RADIOLOGICAL ATLAS OF CHILD ABUSE

RADIOLOGICAL ATLAS OF CHILD ABUSE

AMAKA C OFFIAH
Academic Consultant
Department of Radiology
Great Ormond Street Hospital for Children, London

and

CHRISTINE M HALL
Consultant Paediatric Radiologist
Department of Radiology
Great Ormond Street Hospital for Children, London

Foreword by

JOANNA FAIRHURST
Consultant Paediatric Radiologist
Southampton University Hospitals Trust

Radcliffe Publishing
Oxford • New York

Radcliffe Publishing Ltd
18 Marcham Road
Abingdon
Oxon OX14 1AA
United Kingdom

www.radcliffe-oxford.com

Electronic catalogue and worldwide online ordering facility.

British Library Cataloguing in Publication Data

A catalogue record for this book is available from the British Library.

ISBN-13: 978 1 84619 043 8

Typeset by Pindar NZ, Auckland, New Zealand
Printed and bound by TJ International Ltd, Padstow, Cornwall, UK

Contents

Foreword

Like it or not, as professionals who deal with the care of children, we cannot escape involvement to some degree or other in the field of suspected child abuse. Whether that involvement takes the form of reporting the radiographs of children attending the emergency department or a pathologist called upon to examine a sudden infant death, we have a responsibility to discharge our duty to that child to the best of our ability. To prepare ourselves for this responsibility we need to be fully armed and fully informed. In practical terms this often means accessing information from a variety of sources and using every opportunity which presents itself to gain more experience in this field. The subtlety of the radiological findings compounded by the wide variation in appearance of the developing skeleton frequently leads to a lack of agreement between reporters. This in turn contributes to the atmosphere of stress and uncertainty in what is already an emotionally challenging area of practice.

Thankfully Professor Hall and Dr Offiah have used their extensive experience and exhaustive study of the radiology of child abuse to produce a text which at last fills a significant gap in this field. This volume addresses key issues facing the reporting radiologist both acutely in making a diagnosis and thus identifying a child in need of protection, and subsequently as part of the continued process of child protection proceedings.

The format of this text provides a comprehensive review of key areas such as image production, differential diagnosis and fracture dating, and a detailed illustration of patterns of injury. Each image is enhanced by pertinent learning points that help to consolidate the messages conveyed by the text. It is these pointers, together with the breadth of images and thorough contextual review, that make this atlas unique and ensure that it will provide a lasting contribution to the literature in this field. The atlas will be an invaluable source of reference material that will act as a teaching resource for those new to this area, will consolidate and confirm practice for those professionals already familiar with this field, and will stimulate research into questions which remain unanswered in this arena.

The authors' approach and detailed image analysis make this comprehensive review accessible to all who care for children. In presenting this atlas, Professor Hall and Dr Offiah have enhanced our understanding and provided a major tool with which to help our most vulnerable young patients.

Joanna Fairhurst
Consultant Paediatric Radiologist
Southampton University Hospitals Trust
April 2009

Preface

Which is the lesser error – to make a wrongful diagnosis of physical abuse thus removing an infant from loving carers, or to miss the diagnosis and return a baby to an environment in which episodes of abuse may escalate, culminating in that baby's death? Both scenarios are distinct possibilities; the difficulty with making the diagnosis of abuse (particularly in non-lethal cases) is that no external gold standard exists.

The situation is complicated by the fact that the radiological abnormalities associated with suspected abuse can be extremely subtle. It is well recognised that acute rib fractures are often missed, and there are several normal variants that may be mistaken for fractures. It is therefore important that a paediatric radiologist with experience in dealing with such cases reviews all radiographs obtained as part of a skeletal survey to exclude physical abuse.

The purpose of this atlas is not to turn readers into immediate experts, but rather to offer assistance with initial interpretation of what are often difficult and subtle findings in the emotionally charged environment that frequently exists when child abuse is suspected.

It is hoped that this atlas will be of particular use to radiologists (both in training and at consultant level – specialist or with an interest in paediatric radiology). The atlas may also be useful to those in other specialties including Histopathology and Accident and Emergency.

We have tried to include as many examples of the sorts of difficult cases/normal variants that are encountered in day-to-day practice; however, if readers should come across particularly rare/interesting examples for inclusion in a future edition of this atlas, we should welcome these with gratitude.

Finally, we acknowledge all those who have referred cases to us over the years – without you this atlas would not have been possible.

Amaka C Offiah
Christine M Hall
April 2009

About the authors

Dr Amaka Offiah BSc, MBBS, MRCP, FRCR, PhD graduated from Ahmadu Bello University, Zaria, Nigeria in 1990 and came to England in 1992 following house jobs and National Youth Service. She trained as a radiologist in Sheffield, and joined the Institute of Child Health/Great Ormond Street Hospital in 2000 as a clinical research fellow. In 2005 she was awarded a University of London PhD for her thesis 'Optimisation of the digital radiographic imaging of suspected non-accidental injury'. Her interest lies in the musculoskeletal system, particularly physical child abuse and constitutional bone disorders. She is Chairperson of the Great Ormond Street Child Abuse and Protection Group and serves as an expert witness for the Courts. She is presently an Academic Consultant at Great Ormond Street Hospital for Children, conducting research in the imaging of paediatric musculoskeletal disorders.

Professor Christine Hall MBBS, DMRD, FRCR, MD qualified in 1968 from University College, London. She trained in radiology between 1970 and 1975 at University College Hospital and was appointed Consultant Paediatric Radiologist at Great Ormond Street Hospital in 1975. She held this post until her retirement in March 2008. Her particular interests have included the field of physical child abuse, in relation to which she has frequently appeared as an expert witness to the Courts. She also has a specialist interest in the radiological diagnosis of constitutional bone disorders. She has published almost 200 peer-reviewed papers in addition to many book chapters, two books and an electronic atlas of malformation syndromes and skeletal dysplasias.

Acknowledgement

The authors should like to acknowledge the assistance of Mr Paul Barnard, Department of Medical Illustration, Great Ormond Street Hospital, for his expertise in digitising and annotating the radiographs.

Paul has worked in the Medical Illustration Department for 10 years. Previously he has worked for the National Gallery and Sotheby's and maintains a dedication for archival documentation. In 2005 he gained a Higher National Diploma in Photography and Digital Imaging.

Paul specialises in digitising and cataloguing extensive collections of original flat material including historic literature and early photographic plates, film and prints, and (of course) radiological images. The end use of this material is invariably for online departmental catalogues, on-screen presentations, publications (such as this atlas), and web access.

Paul has worked closely with the authors and the Radiology Department in general for many years. Without his input this atlas would not have been possible. He maintained his patience and humour throughout the production process – together we trawled through hundreds of images (more than once) and yet have managed to remain on speaking terms!

We thank him.

Image production, display and interpretation in child abuse

CHAPTER 1

Evidence-based radiology in child abuse

BACKGROUND

Ambroise Tardieu, a physician in France, first described the findings associated with inflicted childhood injury, in 1860, 35 years before the discovery of X-rays by Wilhelm Conrad Roentgen.[1] However the 'father' of radiological imaging in child abuse must surely be John Caffey, who in 1946 gave us the first radiological description of the findings.[2] In his seminal paper, Caffey described the association of multiple long bone fractures and chronic subdural haematoma in infants. Since that time, the definition of child abuse has been expanded and refined, such that the Child Abuse Prevention and Treatment Act (North America) now states that

> Child abuse and neglect means the physical or mental injury, sexual abuse, negligent treatment, or maltreatment of a child under the age of 18 by a person who is responsible for the child's welfare under circumstances which indicate the child's health or welfare is harmed or threatened thereby.[3]

In summary, there are four major types of abuse: neglect, and physical, sexual and emotional abuse.

The radiologist deals with physical abuse (commonly termed non-accidental injury, but also variously known as the parent–infant traumatic stress or Caffey–Kempe syndrome, inflicted/intentional injury, and the battered or shaken baby/babe syndrome).

Infants and young children are the most vulnerable in terms of fatal injuries resulting from abuse with up to 90% of child abuse and neglect fatalities occurring in those less than five years old, and 41% in those less than a year old.[4] The majority of infants who die following abuse have associated skeletal injuries, usually in the healing phase at the time of their death.[5] In both lethal and non-lethal cases, severe skeletal, neurological and organ damage may exist in the absence of significant clinical/external signs and it is imperative that high-quality radiographs of all bones are obtained.

IMAGING

There is scant evidence in the literature to support specific imaging modalities or views for any given modality. Kemp, *et al.* have performed a systematic review addressing this very issue.[6] For the detection of skeletal injury they advocate a skeletal survey in combination with a nuclear medicine bone scan. They recognise that prospective research is required comparing skeletal surveys with oblique chest views; skeletal surveys with bone scans; skeletal survey plus repeat radiographs in two weeks; and bone scan plus skull and dedicated views of epiphyses and metaphyses.

SKELETAL SURVEY

The radiographs obtained in cases of suspected abuse are collectively known as the skeletal survey. The skeletal survey is the primary investigation of choice for any child under the age of two years where physical abuse is suspected, and once the suspicion has been raised, the full skeletal survey MUST be performed.

In the past, there has been significant variation in the individual radiographs obtained by different Radiology Departments. Thus Offiah and Hall in 2003 showed that of 50 consecutive surveys received by them for a second opinion in suspected abuse, there were 37 different patterns of radiographs obtained.[7] Furthermore, no survey concurred with the British Society of Paediatric Radiologists' (BSPR) guidelines.[8] The study was repeated three years later[9] with more acceptable results (15% of surveys complying with the guidelines).

Some general rules apply.

— The imaging system should be of high quality.
— There should be tight collimation of each anatomical area.
— Additional views should be taken of any known sites of injury, of clinically suspicious sites and of abnormal sites identified on the radiographs. In one series, additional radiographs following a two-week interval increased the detection rate of fractures by 27%.[10] Additional (delayed) radiographs are also of benefit when attempting to date fractures.

Radiographs should be obtained according to the BSPR guidelines[8] (these differ slightly from those of the American College of Radiology (ACR) Standards[11]).

In brief the BSPR guidelines advise the following:

— anteroposterior and left and right oblique radiographs of the chest
— anteroposterior and lateral skull
— anteroposterior limbs (or individual long bones)
— posteroanterior hands
— dorso-plantar feet
— lateral spine including cervical spine
— anteroposterior abdomen to include the pelvis and lower ribs.

A radiologist with paediatric radiology experience, who will be providing a report, should review the skeletal survey for appropriate quality of the images. Double reporting is recommended.

Additional radiographs may be required on an individual basis.

— Coned views of metaphyses.
— Lateral long bone radiographs when a shaft fracture is identified, to evaluate displacement.
— Towne's view of the skull if an occipital injury is suspected either clinically or from the initial radiographs.
— Delayed (limited) skeletal survey (1–2 weeks following the initial survey): to identify additional fractures not initially apparent. These are usually earlier acute rib fractures that may only become apparent once callus develops. Delayed images may also help in the evaluation of the healing process and in dating fractures.
— A skeletal survey on children under the age of two years with the same carers will identify or exclude fractures not apparent on clinical examination.

RADIONUCLIDE BONE SCAN

A bone scan is sometimes advocated as an adjunct to the initial skeletal survey, or as a delayed investigation, to help to identify fractures missed on the radiographic skeletal survey. Until results of a well-designed prospective study are known, the bone scan should not replace an initial skeletal survey. However it may identify missed rib and spinal fractures and sometimes, old virtually healed fractures. Whether or not a radionuclide bone scan is performed will depend on local expertise in performing high quality studies in this difficult age group.

PITFALLS OF A RADIONUCLIDE BONE SCAN

– A scan typically takes of the order of 15 minutes to perform and any movement or incorrect positioning during this time results in poor image quality and the potential for misinterpretation.
– As a consequence of the previous point, it may be necessary to sedate the child.
– Skull fractures do not show increased uptake of isotope.
– All the rapidly growing physes and adjacent metaphyses show increased uptake of isotope. This may give rise to false positives (over-reporting of metaphyseal fractures) or false negatives (under-reporting of metaphyseal fractures).
– Dating fractures is not possible.

CT SCAN
HEAD CT

Because head injury may be occult, it is recommended that computed tomography (CT) of the head is also routinely performed in any child under the age of two with a suspicion of physical abuse.[12] It should be performed on soft tissue and bone window settings. If fractures are identified, reconstruction of images on bony windows may be helpful for court purposes. The head CT should not replace the skull radiographs performed as part of the skeletal survey. It is possible for skull fractures to be missed on CT when they are in the same plane as the tomographic cut. In addition, the width of a skull fracture is traditionally evaluated from the digital/analogue radiographs.

INTRA-ABDOMINAL TRAUMA

Abdominal trauma may be suspected when a child presents with an acute abdomen and other evidence of trauma. Anterior (costochondral) rib fractures (particularly of the lower ribs) may be the result of a direct blow to the epigastrium and have a high association with intra-abdominal injury.[13] Appropriate investigations include ultrasound and CT of the chest and abdomen.

ULTRASOUND/MRI

These other modalities do not form a routine part of the investigation of physical child abuse other than in patient management and in particular, in serious head injuries. In individual cases, soft tissue injuries and periosteal damage may be identified on ultrasound, and magnetic resonance imaging (MRI) has a role in some joint and soft tissue injuries.

POST-MORTEM INVESTIGATIONS

Post-mortem radiographs form an important part of a full forensic investigation into the cause of death of either a sudden unexpected death in infancy (SUDI) or an obvious case of physical abuse of an infant or child. It is recommended that a full skeletal survey as detailed above be undertaken before the start of the post-mortem examination. A forensic pathologist – preferably a paediatric pathologist – should perform the post-mortem according to published guidelines.[14] Selected areas of the skeleton thought to show evidence of injury from the skeletal survey and post-mortem examination may then be resected and decalcified for further specimen radiography and histology. This is the most rigorous approach to identifying and dating individual injuries. Fracture dating cannot be precise with either a radiological or pathological approach alone. Both disciplines should be regarded as complementary to each other. In general, histology gives more precise dating in the first week following a fracture, but radiographic evaluation is more reliable after that time.

For further details including technical parameters of the imaging system and qualifications of involved personnel, the interested reader is referred to the British Society of Paediatric Radiologists' standard for skeletal surveys in suspected abuse[8] and the American College of Radiology practice guidelines for skeletal surveys in children.[11]

COMPUTED/DIGITAL VS ANALOGUE RADIOGRAPHY

Computed radiography (CR), also known as storage phosphor radiography was first introduced in the early 1980s.[15] It is a form of digital imaging increasing in popularity because of advances in technology (picture archiving and communication systems – PACS) allowing for 'filmless' departments. The system consists of two major components: (1) a reusable laser-stimulated luminescent phosphor imaging plate and (2) a scanning and recording mechanism.[16] The phosphor plate is sensitive to X-rays but relatively insensitive to light. While expensive, it can be reused several thousand times.[17]

Digital radiography (DR) systems (whether direct or indirect) have no need for an imaging plate as images are sent directly to a computer for processing. Image quality is better than that obtained with CR or traditional film/screen systems.[18]

The techniques have several practical advantages over conventional film-screen radiography, including economic and ergonomic.[19] In terms of technical efficacy, there is reduced spatial, but increased contrast resolution.[20] These differences are detectable clinically as reduced visibility of cortex and trabecular markings (spatial resolution) and increased visibility of soft tissues (contrast resolution) when interpreting CR compared to film screen radiographs of the paediatric lateral spine.[21]

CR systems have the ability to produce radiographs of almost constant density regardless of exposure parameters.[20] There is therefore potential for dose reduction. However, although film density remains constant, in clinical practice dose reduction is limited by an increase in quantum mottle. This may have significant (not as yet quantified) effects on the observer's ability to visualise the subtle fractures of abuse.

Digital systems allow (limited) post processing. When used optimally post processing improves visualisation of pathology, and allows both bone and soft tissue detail (for example) to be clearly visualised on the same radiograph. Techniques include magnification, grey-scale, contrast, brightness, non-linear grey-scale enhancement, non-linear unsharp masking (edge-enhancement) and single or dual exposure energy subtraction.

In the case of physical abuse, it has been shown that neither post processing parameters (magnification and edge enhancement) nor method of digital image display (i.e., whether radiographs were printed or viewed from a monitor) affect the diagnostic accuracy of individual observers.[22] Furthermore there is significant variability in diagnostic accuracy between observers.

To conclude, with digital radiography systems, emphasis should be placed on observer training and experience rather than image display and post processing techniques.

INDIVIDUAL INJURIES

Depending on the age of the study population, an estimated 10% to 70% of physically abused children manifest some form of skeletal trauma.[23-6] Furthermore, fractures are second only to soft tissue injury as the commonest presentation of physical child abuse.[27]

SOFT TISSUE INJURY

Although multiple bruising is the commonest presenting feature in (physically) abused children,[27] it is also a common finding in the normal non-abused infant and child. In one study of accidental fractures, Mathew, *et al.* found that 91% of children had no associated bruising at presentation, and most (72%) remained without evidence of bruising in the first week after their injury.[28] Carpenter examined 177 six to twelve month old babies presenting routinely to child health clinics, and found a prevalence rate of 12% for (presumed) accidental bruises.[29] This is comparable to the prevalence of 12.5% observed by Roberton, *et al.* in a study on 62 babies aged three to nine months old.[30] Accidental bruising is most often found on the face and head, on the front of the trunk and over bony prominences. All accidental lower limb bruising occurs in mobile children. The incidence of bruising in children increases significantly with increasing mobility.[29] In contrast, multiple bruises of different ages, bruises over soft sites (e.g., the cheeks), and lower limb bruising in a non-mobile infant are all suggestive of abuse.[29,31] Some soft tissue injuries are obviously non-accidental, e.g., cigarette burns and bite marks.

Even minor injury to the soft tissues results in haemorrhage and inflammatory exudate. This manifests on radiographs as obliteration of the normal radiolucency of the superficial and deep soft tissue planes. There may also be displacement of the fat planes around the site of injury.[32] Bruising may or may not be associated with underlying bony injury.[33] Conversely severe skeletal injuries involving acceleration-deceleration forces alone may occur in the absence of visible signs of injury.[34] This means that when physical abuse is suspected, the entire skeletal survey must be performed regardless of the presence or absence of bruising. Closer scrutiny and a lower threshold for repeating dedicated views of bones underlying clinical bruising may increase the detection rate of skeletal injury.

Generally speaking, bruising is not a radiological diagnosis, although reports exist describing radiological features such as calcified haematomas in older children,[35] as well as a case of so called 'necklace calcification' in the soft tissues of the neck presumed due to fat necrosis following strangulation.[36] The major benefit in recognising the radiological features of soft tissue injury is that they help to determine the age of the fracture particularly those affecting the shafts of the long bones. There is a gradual increase in the size of swelling overlying the site of the fracture over the course of the first three to four days after a fracture has been sustained. This is accompanied by loss of definition of the soft tissue planes, initially at the site of the fracture, but over the course of the four days after a fracture, this extends up and down the limb away from the fracture site. Thereafter the swelling gradually subsides and generally has resolved by seven to ten days after the fracture has occurred. These changes in the soft tissues are seen before there is evidence of bony healing.

METAPHYSEAL FRACTURES

The reported incidence of metaphyseal fractures in physical abuse ranges from 11% to 53%.[23,37-9] Although less common than diaphyseal fractures,[38,40,41] metaphyseal fractures are the most specific single sign of physical abuse.[40,42,43] They occur most commonly in the lower limbs around the knees and ankles,[31] but are also seen around the other joints of the upper and lower limbs.[44]

Metaphyseal fractures are variously known as metaphyseal infractions, avulsion fractures and metaphyseal spurs. Kleinman suggests they be referred to as classical metaphyseal lesions (CML).[45] For the sake of consistency, the term 'CML' has been adopted in the remainder of this text.

The CML was originally thought to represent an avulsion injury of the periphery of the metaphysis.[46] However, Kleinman, *et al.*[8,47–51] have characterised these lesions histologically, and thus explained their radiological appearances and likely mechanism of injury. In brief, the CML is a series of planar microfractures through the most immature portion of the metaphyseal primary spongiosa. The fracture line extends in a planar fashion towards the periphery (cortex) of the bone. As it does so, it veers away from the physis (growth plate) undercutting a bony peripheral segment that encompasses the subperiosteal bone collar. As a consequence, the peripheral bony fragment(s) will be thicker than the central portion.

Traditionally the CML has been divided into two types based on radiological appearance; namely 'corner' and 'bucket-handle' fractures.[40] However these are in fact the same lesion. The radiological appearance depends on the radiographic projection.[45] When imaged with the beam at 90° to the long axis of the diaphysis (in the same plane as the physis), the CML has a corner fracture configuration. The relatively thick peripheral portion of the fracture is seen end-on as a somewhat discrete triangular fragment. A bucket-handle appearance of the fracture results from imaging the same lesion with beam angulation (more or less than 90°). In this instance, beam angulation throws the fractured metaphysis off the diaphysis, and it is seen as a curvilinear radiodensity.

Metaphyseal lesions occur as a result of direct shearing or twisting forces, and are also said to occur during shaking when indirect acceleration-deceleration forces are applied to the infant's limbs.[31,41,45]

DIAPHYSEAL FRACTURES

Although less specific for abuse, diaphyseal fractures are four times commoner than the CML of physical abuse.[38,40] Multiple fractures of the shafts of the long bones are highly suspicious.[52] Apart from bruising, the most common initial presentation of abuse is an isolated diaphyseal fracture.[38,53,54] Of the fracture types, transverse fractures are the commonest.[31,55] The middle (50%) and distal third (41%) locations are the most prominent sites of long bone fracture.[53] Extremity fractures have been shown to occur at a younger age than skull fractures in a cohort of patients under a year old.[56]

The most commonly fractured bone varies from series to series, with the tibia, femur and humerus being variously cited.[23,25–7,38,53,57] In the most recent series,[39] the commonest site of an isolated long bone fracture was the humerus (including one metaphyseal fracture) followed by the femur (including two metaphyseal fractures).

Humerus In young children, a humeral shaft fracture rarely occurs in accidental injury and has a high association with abuse.[27,37,53] Physical abuse should be considered in all children less than 15 months old with humeral fractures, including those children with supracondylar fractures.[58]

Tibia A tibial shaft fracture in a non-ambulatory child is highly suspicious of abuse, particularly when an inappropriate history is given.[52] Although Loder and Bookout[38] reported the tibia as the commonest long bone to be fractured in abuse, it must be emphasised that two-thirds of these tibial fractures were in fact metaphyseal and not diaphyseal. Toddler's fractures (hairline spiral fractures of the tibial shaft) occur in the ambulant child. Their recognition is important to avoid the over-diagnosis of physical abuse.[31]

Femur Like tibial fractures, femoral fractures in the non-ambulant child are highly suspicious of physical abuse. Of course ambulant children may also be abused, hence the importance of a detailed history.[59–61] Many practitioners believe spiral fractures to be pathognomonic of physical abuse.[55] This is not the case, as no single type or site of fracture is significantly more associated with or characteristic of physical abuse.[31] Beals and Tufts[60] suggest that subtrochanteric femoral fractures are more common in non-accidental than accidental injury in children. This opinion is not supported by the work of Scherl, *et al.*[55] In fact these authors concluded that because spiral fractures are viewed as particularly suspicious, care must be taken not to miss cases of physical abuse in children with transverse fractures.

Radius/Ulna Although they are fractured commonly in accidental trauma, the radius and ulna are the least fractured long bones in child physical abuse.[25–7,38,53,57]

Findings suggestive of physical abuse were summarised by Leventhal, *et al.*,[62] and include:

— fractures in children whose carers give a history of behavioural change in the child, but no accidental event, or a minor fall not consistent with the severity of the sustained injury
— fractures of the radius and ulna, tibia and fibula, or femur in children less than a year old
— mid shaft or metaphyseal fractures of the humerus.

Mechanisms of injury include direct trauma (in an older child attempting to fend off a blow), inappropriate pulling (causing the bone to fracture under the weight of the suspended struggling child (infant), an awkward fall (as the child (infant) is thrown or pushed away), or a twisting force.[11,31,41] By their nature, spiral fractures imply a twisting force, and are therefore highly suggestive of abuse.[37,41] Care must be taken when attributing a spiral fracture to physical abuse – history, patient age and development, fracture age, and the presence of other injuries must all be taken into consideration to reduce the risk of over or under diagnosis.[63]

SKULL FRACTURES

Skull fractures are the commonest[38,62] or second most common[52] skeletal injury in cases of physical abuse, depending on case selection. They are said to be more frequent in non-accidental than in accidental injury.[43] This is particularly true of the younger child – 3% of skull fractures in one series of patients less than 13 years of age were due to child physical abuse,[64] compared to 33% in a group of children less than two years of age.[65] In another study of 189 battered children, skull fractures were the only fracture type more likely to be present in children aged less than a year compared to older children.[53]

A fall out of bed is a rare cause of skull fracture.[66,67] Simple linear fractures occur from a height of three to five and a half feet (i.e., from domestic falls), while more complex (accidental) fractures occur from a height of six or more feet.[68] The majority of stairway injuries are relatively insignificant (because they consist of a series of low height, low impact falls). Although falls may be associated with severe injury,[69] the presence of multiple sites of injury following an alleged fall down a flight of stairs should be viewed with more suspicion than should a solitary skull fracture.[70]

Most skull fractures occurring in cases of physical abuse cannot on their own be differentiated from those occurring in accidental trauma, and there is no single appearance that is pathognomonic of abuse.[35] There are some features however which favour a diagnosis of physical abuse, these include non-parietal fractures; complex fractures (especially if both sides are affected); multiple fractures; fractures equal to or greater than 4 mm in width;

growing fractures; depressed fractures (especially occipital); and fractures associated with intracranial injury.[64,65]

It must be remembered that a skull fracture crossing a suture to involve more than one bone may be the result of a single blow with the fracture line radiating in both directions from the single impact site.[63] This occurrence is most frequent in the parietal bones, although occasionally the occiput may be involved.

The absence of a skull fracture does not exclude significant intracranial injury.[31] It has been recommended that following blunt trauma, skull radiography should be performed in children older than two years of age only if physical abuse is suspected. It may also be performed to confirm the presence of a depressed fracture. On the other hand, skull radiography should be performed in all children less than two years old because of the higher likelihood of abuse in this group.[71] In suspected physical abuse, even in the absence of neurological signs, intracranial injury should be excluded by cross-sectional imaging whenever the radiograph confirms a skull fracture.[72] It has recently been advocated that cross-sectional neurological imaging be performed routinely in cases of suspected physical abuse,[12] and it is now part of the routine protocol in many departments in the United Kingdom.

RIB FRACTURES

Ninety per cent of abuse-related rib fractures occur in children less than two years of age.[40] The presence of multiple rib injuries adds considerably to the radiologist's confidence in making a diagnosis of abuse. They were not mentioned in Caffey's original description of the association between long bone fractures and subdural haematomas,[2] but with the expansion of the radiological phenotype of child abuse, their importance was soon recognised.[73,74]

The ribs of infants and young children are relatively pliable, and therefore with normal day-to-day handling of the child, fractures at this site should be uncommon.[68] Any of the 12 ribs may be fractured, and individual ribs may fracture anywhere along their arc depending on the mechanism of the inflicted injury. A compressive squeezing force in the anteroposterior (front-to-back) direction results in lateral rib fractures, and in the lateral (side-to-side) direction produces anterior or posterior fractures. Rib fractures in this age group may also occur as a result of accidental trauma (following notable trauma such as a road traffic accident), occasionally following cardiopulmonary resuscitation (CPR), bone fragility, birth trauma, chest physiotherapy and severe coughing.[75-8] However the occurrence of rib fractures due to these causes in infants is very uncommon.

Thomas[79] reviewed 10 000 infants, and found rib fractures (from any cause, including some cases of abuse) in only 25. Others[80] have failed to demonstrate rib fractures in a large cohort (greater than 13 000) of live births. Furthermore post-mortem radiological and histological examination failed to demonstrate a single rib fracture in a cohort of 91 patients under a year old after failed cardiopulmonary resuscitation.[81]

In summary, child physical abuse must always be considered in an infant found to have rib fractures.

The reported incidence of rib fractures in physical abuse ranges from 5% to 29%.[25,37-9,53] It has been said that these figures probably represent an underestimate[68] with 80% of rib fractures being occult.[40] There are at least two reasons for the difficulties in radiographic identification of rib fractures. Firstly the X-ray beam may not align with the fracture line. Furthermore overlapping structures may easily obscure the fracture line (particularly in the acute phase).[41] Kleinman, et al.[82] reported that of 84 rib fractures demonstrated on post-mortem histopathology studies, only 30 (36%) were visible on the original skeletal survey. It is also known that high-detail post-mortem radiography of dissected ribs allows visualisation of fractures not visible on pre-dissection radiographs. This is illustrated in Plates 3.12 and 3.13. These disturbing findings perhaps explain the advice given by the BSPR[8] to routinely perform left and right oblique projections of the rib cage in addition to the anteroposterior chest radiograph as part of the skeletal survey in suspected physical abuse.

Ng and Hall[13] reported a relationship between fractures of the anterior ends (costo-chondral junctions) of the lower ribs (6th–9th) and intra-abdominal visceral injury. These fractures were difficult to visualise, were equated to the 'bucket handle' CML, and were associated with major abdominal visceral trauma.

Boal has published results on her analysis of 910 cases referred over 13 years. Of 1463 rib fractures in abused children, 12% occurred at the costochondral junction, 0% in children thought not to have been abused and 15% in those in whom a definite distinction between abuse and other cause could not be made.[63]

SUBPERIOSTEAL NEW BONE FORMATION

Subperiosteal new bone formation (SPNBF) may be seen in physical abuse in two contexts:
— as a normal response to fracture healing
— in the absence of a fracture, as a radiological feature of abuse (periosteal trauma).

The radiological evidence of healing fractures is dealt with later, while isolated SPNBF as a feature of abuse is discussed below.

Caffey[2] described the finding in his seminal paper, and it has since been demonstrated to be relatively common in abused children.[54]

The pathological finding is haemorrhage causing the osteogenic layer of periosteum to be stripped from the underlying cortex. The osteogenic layer of periosteum adheres tightly to the metaphyses and epiphyses, and more loosely to the diaphyses of bones. As a result, collections of subperiosteal blood are of maximum diameter along the shafts and taper towards the ends (except in the case of massive haemorrhage or repetitive trauma).[45,52,68]

Tractional and torsional forces on the periosteum as a result of rough gripping and twisting or pulling of an extremity, was initially felt to be the mechanism of causation of SPNBF. Some workers also feel that SPNBF can occur following acceleration-deceleration forces.[31,45,68]

SPNBF is not specific to physical abuse. It may be seen as a result of infectious, trau-matic, metabolic and neoplastic disease and Caffey's disease. Another important differential diagnosis to consider is benign periosteal reaction, which occurs physiologically and was initially described in infants between the ages of six weeks and six months.[31] It has since been shown that physiological SPNBF most frequently involves the femur or tibia, is usu-ally symmetrical, never extends to the metaphysis, is very rarely greater than 2 mm thick, and is commonest between the ages of one and four months.[83]

As with many other fractures in physical abuse, there may or may not be soft tissue evidence of injury. Radiologically, SPNBF can be easily overlooked, as it may appear only as a faint haziness/irregularity of the affected cortex. In other instances it may be seen as a thin layer of bone separated from the underlying cortex by a narrow radiolucent interval.[45] High-quality radiographs, and multiple and coned views may be required for confident diagnosis or exclusion of SPNBF. The radiographic bone changes represent a healing response to trauma and are only visible about seven days after the injury has occurred.

SPNBF may occur in isolation in physical abuse. However its detection should prompt close scrutiny of the underlying bone to exclude a subtle hairline fracture. This should include projections at right angles to each other, as a hairline fracture may be invisible on one view alone. Once again the need for high-quality examinations cannot be overstated.

LESS COMMON FRACTURES WITH HIGH SPECIFICITY FOR PHYSICAL ABUSE

These include the following:
- axial skeleton: vertebral body, superior pubic ramus
- appendicular skeleton: acromion and body of scapula, metacarpals, metatarsals, epiphyseal fracture/dislocations of upper and lower limb.

RADIOLOGICAL DATING OF FRACTURES

It has been said that in making a diagnosis of physical abuse, the single most important factor is the relationship between the alleged timing of the injury and the radiographic appearance of that injury.[84] However, it may be argued that the single most important factor is in fact the multiplicity of injuries, and that fracture age becomes more important as the number of fractures detected decreases. This by no means belittles the role played by the radiographic dating of fractures in the diagnosis of abuse, as evidenced by the fact that in a recent publication it was recorded that an isolated long bone fracture was seen in 89 of 467 (19%) children with suspected physical abuse.[39] The correct dating of injuries is also of importance to the courts when establishing culpability.

The radiographic changes parallel the histopathological changes; however, it should be noted that there is a significant subjective element to fracture dating by either discipline, and not all radiologists would agree with the time sequence as described.

When a fracture is apparent on radiographs, the presence of significant soft tissue swelling with loss of the normal fat planes informs the radiologist that the injury is recent, probably within the preceding seven (and certainly within the preceding ten) days.

SPNBF is seen on radiographs only once calcification has begun (i.e., about seven to ten days after the fracture has been sustained). Repetitive injury to a non-immobilised fracture as may be seen in physical abuse, leads to further subperiosteal haemorrhage and subsequent exuberant callus formation.[52] It should be noted that SPNBF might not be seen in the healing process of CML,[84] skull, or vertebral fractures.

Fracture margins An acute fracture has well-defined sharp margins. This appearance is present for about seven to ten days after a fracture has occurred. In the early stages of fracture repair, macrophages begin to resorb non-viable tissues including the ends of the affected bone. Radiographically this corresponds to a loss of definition of the fracture margins, with apparent widening of the fracture gap after about seven days. This is the only reliable means by which the CML can be dated.[84]

Soft callus The laying down and calcification of osteoid is visible on radiographs as a subtle increase in density around the fracture site. At this stage the fracture line is still discernible. This is a gradual and ongoing process from about one to six weeks.

This is first seen about seven to ten days after a fracture has been sustained and gradually increases in volume and density.

Hard callus The complete conversion of woven to lamellar bridging bone marks the stable union of the fracture. Radiographically this is evidenced by definite sclerosis around the fracture and consolidation of the callus. By this stage the fracture line may or may not be discernible. The fracture line usually disappears about six to eight weeks after a fracture has occurred.

Remodelling The variability in duration of this phase means that it is not a reliable radiological method of dating fractures. By this stage the acute healing phase is over and the fracture line is not discernable. In undisplaced fractures of long bones and ribs the remodelling process is more or less complete by twelve weeks after a fracture.

The radiologist should be aware that the healing of fractures is dependent on many variables including patient age, affected bone, degree of displacement, presence of re-fracturing, force of injury, fixation and immobilisation of the affected fragments, etc.

There are some exceptions to the generalisations given above.

Firstly, unless the adjacent periosteum is damaged, SPNBF does not occur with the healing of CMLs. In such cases the most reliable means by which these fractures can be dated is by assessment of the fracture line.[84] It is unusual to see soft tissue changes associated with CMLs. Undisplaced CMLs have usually healed radiographically by consolidation to the adjacent bone by four weeks after they were sustained. Kleinman, *et al.*[85] correlated radiological with histopathological changes of CMLs in a retrospective analysis of 13 distal tibial CMLs. Nine of these fractures were shown histologically to be in a healing phase, and all nine were associated with a focal radiolucent extension from the growth plate into the metaphysis. The authors imply that with knowledge of the relative growth rates of various bones, the minimum age of a metaphyseal fracture can be calculated based on the depth of the radiolucency into the metaphysis.

Secondly, skull fractures do not demonstrate the radiological features listed. The associated scalp swelling may help to date acute fractures, but literature on this topic is limited. Swelling is best evaluated on bone window settings of the CT head scan.

Thirdly, rib fractures are difficult to detect radiographically, particularly in the acute phase. SPNBF may not be differentiated from overlying pulmonary vascular markings. Indeed SPNBF may not develop, particularly with anterior costochondral rib fractures.[83,86] This is similar to the healing pattern of CMLs, with which they are analogous. The subsequent formation of callus helps to identify and date previously unidentified fractures or suspicious areas. In one study, repeat radiographs approximately two weeks after the initial ones increased the pick-up of fractures by 27%, and yielded important information regarding age of fracture in 19% of 70 previously detected fractures. The majority of these fractures were rib fractures and CMLs.[20] Follow-up surveys might therefore be recommended in suspicious cases to provide a more accurate assessment of bony injury. In some institutions follow-up surveys form part of the routine skeletal survey. The BSPR standard[8] does not address this issue.

A recent systematic review of studies related to fracture dating performed between 1966 and 2004 found only three suitable for inclusion.[87] The conclusion was that there is an urgent need for research to validate the criteria used in the radiological dating of fractures in children less than five years.

Although the radiological dating of fractures is occasionally described as more of an art than a science, it does in fact require considerable experience of the various appearances of fracture healing in infants.

It is advised that radiologists date fractures with caution, and always cite a range rather than a specific age for each injury identified.

DIFFERENTIAL DIAGNOSIS

There are a number of pathological conditions and normal variants that may be misdiagnosed as abuse. Particularly in the case of pathology, there may be other radiological and/or clinical findings that help in reaching the diagnosis.

A definite diagnosis may not always be reached, and on occasion it is beneficial to perform follow up radiographs in 14 days, particularly in the case of suspected normal variants. A fracture evolves with healing, whereas a normal variant remains unchanged (over the 14-day time period).

The importance of a detailed history (including mechanism of injury) cannot be over-emphasised, as often this is the only way of distinguishing accidental from non-accidental trauma.

SUMMARY

This chapter has consisted of a review of the current literature.

There are many areas in which further prospective research is required; nevertheless, some important conclusions can be reached.

— All infants and children less than two years of age who are suspected of being physically abused should have a skeletal survey performed.
— The skeletal survey should be performed according to the BSPR guidelines.[8]
— The skeletal survey should routinely include a CT of the brain.
— All imaging should be reviewed by paediatric radiologists with experience of cases of suspected abuse.
— Until more research has been carried out, fractures should be dated with caution. A range of dates should be cited.
— The current belief is that CMLs may be caused by either direct tractional/torsional forces or by the acceleration-deceleration forces associated with violent shaking.
— Anterior fractures of the lower ribs are commonly associated with intra-abdominal injury.
— Fractures will evolve with time (over the course of two weeks); normal variants will not – and are usually bilateral and symmetrical.
— Physiological periosteal reaction is symmetrical and does not extend to the metaphyseal regions of the bones.
— A significant number of acute rib fractures may be missed on the initial chest radiographs, and delayed radiographs (10–14 days) are advocated.

Skeletal injuries in child abuse

CHAPTER 2

Skull

Skull fractures result from a direct impact of the head against a hard object or surface. Accidental falls under the force of gravity will result in the infant's head, because of its disproportionately large size and weight, impacting the floor first. In infants there needs to be a history of an accident of sufficient magnitude to account for a fracture. The vast majority of domestic falls of up to five feet, solely under the force of gravity do not result in a skull fracture. Rare cases are reported of fractures occurring from low falls. Any force added to the force of gravity increases the likelihood of a fracture occurring. For example this may occur when a carer falls while carrying the infant. In this situation there is the height of the fall (gravity) together with the forward momentum and propulsive force exerted by the adult.

PATTERNS OF SKULL FRACTURES
— A linear, hairline, unilateral parietal fracture is the commonest type of skull fracture seen either as a result of accidental or abusive trauma.
— Other fracture types indicate that forces have occurred that are greater than those generated following a simple fall. They may be more suggestive of abusive physical trauma but need to be put into the context of the history.
  • A fracture crossing a suture line (more than one skull bone fractured). Fractures may travel along the sutures for a short distance and therefore a single impact may result in discontinuous fractures across a suture affecting two bones. Sometimes symmetrical fractures may be present affecting both parietal bones, but not crossing or involving the sagittal suture. These may be the result of two separate impacts, with a higher specificity for abuse, or the result of a single crushing force applied simultaneously to both sides of the head (for example standing on the head of the infant).
  • Wide fractures are those equal to or greater than 4 mm in width measured on the skull radiographs, NOT from CT images of the head.
  • Fissured, branching or stellate fractures. These are more likely to occur following an impact against an object with a relatively small surface area, rather than a flat surface.
  • Depressed fractures. An uncommon type of depressed fracture is the 'ping-pong' fracture in which there is a saucer-shaped depression of the convexity, often with a short fracture line in the centre of the concavity. These should not be confused with the extrinsic concave depression(s) seen as a result of intrauterine moulding and associated with oligohydramnios.
  • Growing fractures are those, which over time, carry on increasing in width. They result from separation of the fracture by the leptomeninges.
  • Fractures not involving the parietal bones, especially occipital fractures.

Soft tissue swelling usually becomes apparent overlying the position of a skull fracture as a combination of the direct effect of the impact and bleeding from the site of the fracture. The swelling may be immediately obvious, or may gradually develop over the course of several hours or days. The swelling becomes maximal and then gradually decreases, the whole process taking 7–10 days. Swelling may initially be identified from the feeling of a soft or boggy sensation on handling the infant's head during bathing or dressing. The time at which the swelling is noted by carers is extremely variable and will depend upon:

— the speed with which the swelling develops
— the carers' observational abilities
— the thickness of the infant's hair
— outer clothing.

SKULL FRACTURE HEALING AND DATING

Skull fractures heal by gradual apposition and fibrous union of the fracture margins over a variable period of time. In the first week or two, the edges of the fracture appear clearly defined and gradually there is then loss of definition of the fracture margins. These appearances may remain the same for weeks or even months after the fracture has occurred and therefore are not helpful in dating a skull fracture. Soft tissue swelling (as identified on soft tissue windows of CT rather than on radiographs), reliably indicates that the fracture is recent. This means that the fracture has occurred within the previous 7–10 day period. CT soft tissue swelling will be apparent even when this is not clinically appreciated. Any associated intracranial injuries may also be helpful in dating a traumatic head injury, assuming that they have occurred on the same occasion as the impact injury causing the fracture. Any skull fracture may be associated with subarachnoid or subdural bleeding directly under the site of the fracture. The impact injury may also result in other more serious intracranial injuries. This is the province of a specialist paediatric neuroradiologist.

EFFECT OF A SKULL FRACTURE

The effects are extremely variable and the severity depends on any associated intracranial injuries resulting either from the impact itself or an associated shaking episode.

— The majority of accidental skull fractures are not associated with intracranial trauma and result in pain at the time the fracture occurs and minor tenderness on direct palpation over the site of the fracture for hours or days afterwards.
— Soft tissue swelling may be apparent for about ten days after the fracture is sustained.
— More serious effects resulting from intracranial injury may range from mild concussion with drowsiness and vomiting to unconsciousness, respiratory arrest and death.

DIFFERENTIAL DIAGNOSIS

— Accidental trauma. This requires the careful evaluation of the history given in relation to the severity and type of injury sustained. The history should be consistent over time and between any witnesses of the injury. Evidence of further injury would detract from the diagnosis of accidental trauma.
— Normal variant findings include fissures and accessory sutures and these may be misinterpreted as fractures. Persistent membranous fissures are a common feature of the young infant's skull. They gradually ossify with continued growth of the skull over weeks or months. Radiographically they appear as short (1–2 cm), tapering, radiolucent lines arising from and at right angles to, the sagittal or lambdoid sutures. Accessory sutures are most commonly present in the lambdoid bone. They are almost always bilaterally symmetrical and lack the clear-cut appearance and parallelism of fracture

lines. Larger intrasutural or wormian bones may be present in the lambdoid suture and result in confusion with fractures. Wormian bones are present at birth and remain visible throughout childhood. Up to ten wormian bones are considered a normal variant finding.

— Cephalhaematomas may occur during delivery, especially following ventouse extraction. A rim of calcification may develop in the haematoma, or they may exert a compression effect and give rise to a cystic appearance in the vault, which may be mistaken for a depressed fracture.

— A 'ping-pong' fracture may mistakenly be interpreted as the result of compression from faulty intra-uterine packing due to oligohydramnios, or vice versa the compression may be interpreted as a fracture.

2.1 SIMPLE LINEAR (HAIRLINE) PARIETAL FRACTURE

Age of fracture: Less than 10 days (soft tissue swelling on CT – arrowhead)

Degree of force: Moderate (simple fracture, <4 mm wide)

Mechanism: Simple/domestic fall

Height of fall: 3.5 to 5 feet

General prevalence: Common

Prevalence in abuse: Common (7%–30%)

Specificity for abuse: Low (commonest fracture in both accidental injury and physical abuse)

➥ Whenever possible, obtain lateral radiograph with side of soft tissue swelling/clinical abnormality closest to imaging plate.
➥ CT may demonstrate soft tissue swelling that is not clinically detectable.
➥ The width of skull fractures is determined from radiographs and NOT from CT scans (original studies[64] measured fracture width from radiographs).

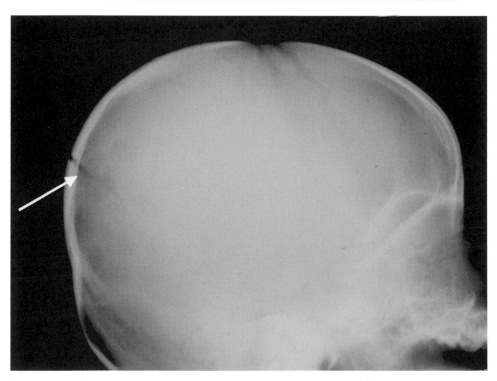

A: Lateral skull

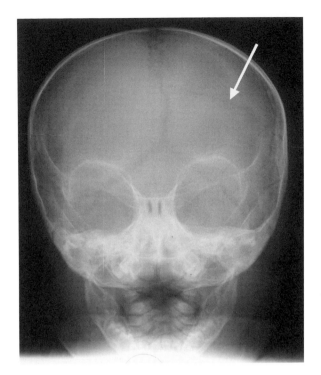

B: AP skull

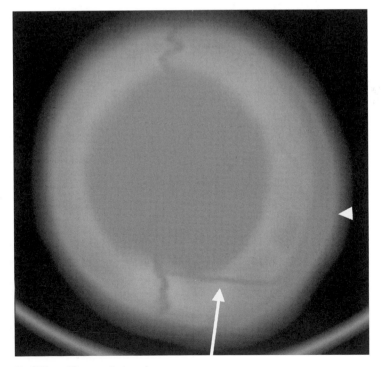

C: CT head (bony windows)

2.2 SIMPLE LINEAR (HAIRLINE) PARIETAL FRACTURE

Age of fracture:	Less than 10 days (soft tissue swelling on CT – arrowhead)
Degree of force:	Moderate (simple fracture, <4 mm wide)
Mechanism:	Simple/domestic fall
Height of fall:	3.5 to 5 feet
Prevalence in abuse:	Common (7%–30%)
Specificity for abuse:	Low (commonest fracture in both accidental injury and physical abuse)

➥ Depending on the angle of the tomographic cut relative to the fracture, CT may miss skull fractures. In this example, only the anterior part of the fracture adjacent to the right coronal suture was demonstrable by CT (arrow).

➥ *See* Plate 2.9.

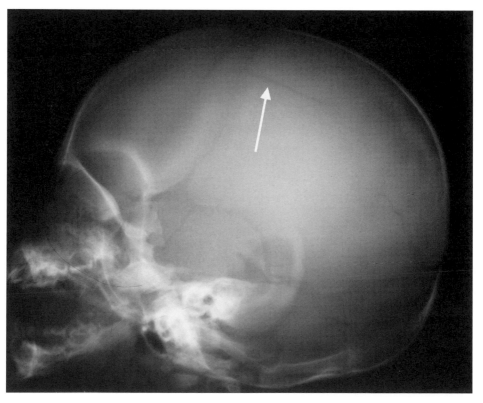

A: Lateral skull

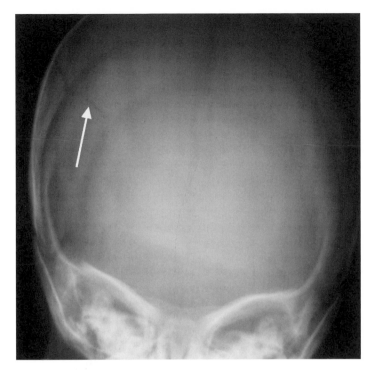

B: AP skull

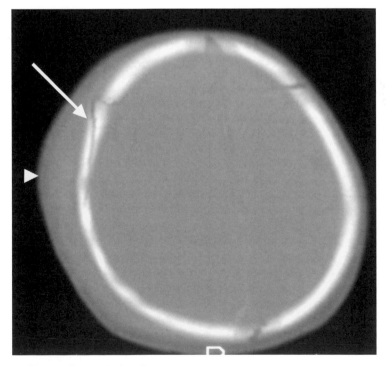

C: CT head (bony windows)

2.3 SIMPLE LINEAR (HAIRLINE) OCCIPITAL FRACTURE

Age of fracture:	Uncertain (in the absence of soft tissue swelling, skull fractures cannot be reliably dated)
Degree of force:	Moderately severe (simple fracture, <4 mm wide, involves the occiput)
Mechanism:	Fall plus gravity
Height of fall:	3.5 to 5 feet
Prevalence in abuse:	Common (7%–30%)
Specificity for abuse:	Moderate (non-parietal location)

➡ Obtain a Towne's projection if an occipital fracture is suspected.

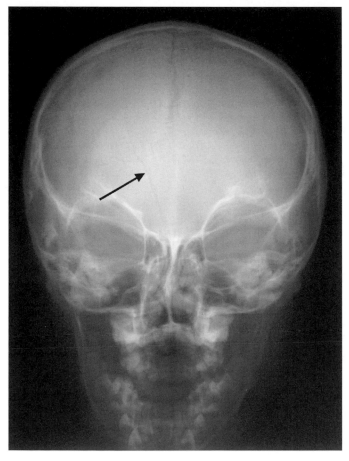

A: AP skull

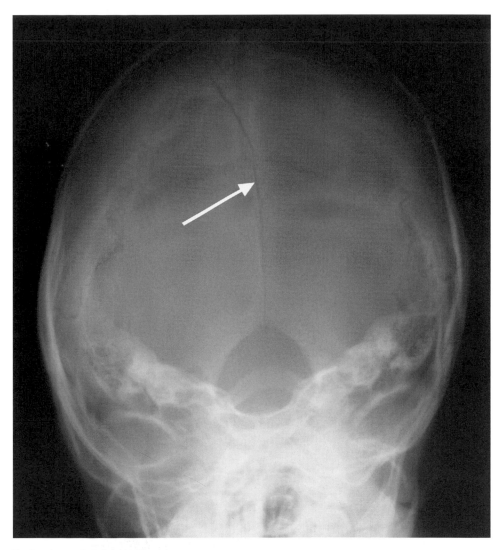

B: Fronto-occipital projection

2.4 SIMPLE LINEAR (HAIRLINE) OCCIPITAL FRACTURE

Age of fracture:	<8 days (the patient is an 8-day-old neonate)
Degree of force:	Severe (branching fracture, involves the occiput)
Mechanism:	Fall plus gravity
Height of fall:	>6 feet
Prevalence in abuse:	Common (7%–30%)
Specificity for abuse:	High (non-parietal location, age of patient, absent history)

➥ Normal vaginal delivery in the absence of instrumentation will not lead to a skull fracture.
➥ Ventouse delivery is unlikely to lead to a skull fracture.
➥ Forceps delivery may lead to fractures, usually of the parietal bone(s).

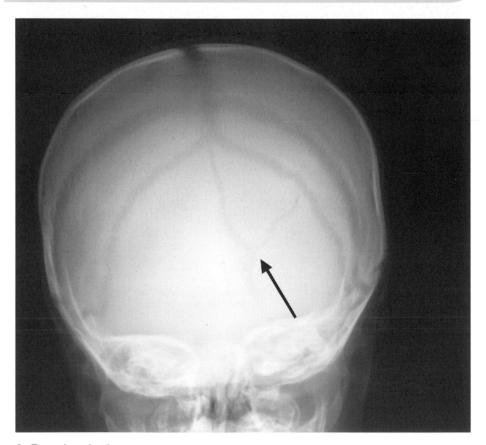

A: Towne's projection

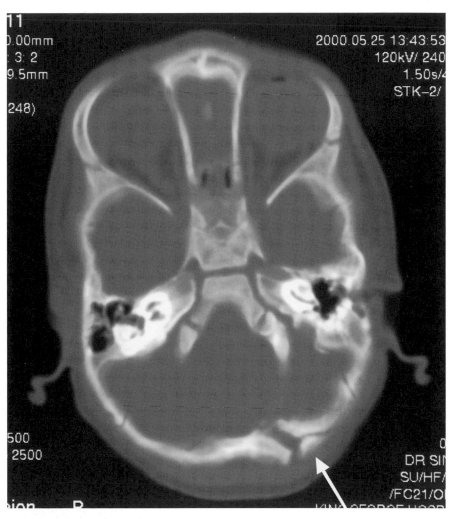

B: CT head (bony windows)

2.5 COMPLEX BILATERAL SKULL FRACTURES

Age of fractures: Uncertain (soft tissue swelling not apparent)

Degree of force: Severe (complex fractures, >4 mm wide, cross sutures to involve all bones, depressed fragments)

Mechanism: Several impacts to both sides of the head or crushing forces

Height of fall: >6 feet or equivalent forces

Prevalence in abuse: Common (7%–30%)

Specificity for abuse: High (in the absence of an acceptable history)

➥ A single impact may result in a discontinuous fracture crossing a suture; however, the complex fractures illustrated here will have resulted from more than one impact or crushing force.

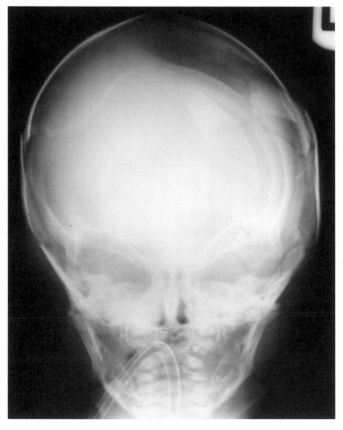

A: Patient 1: AP skull

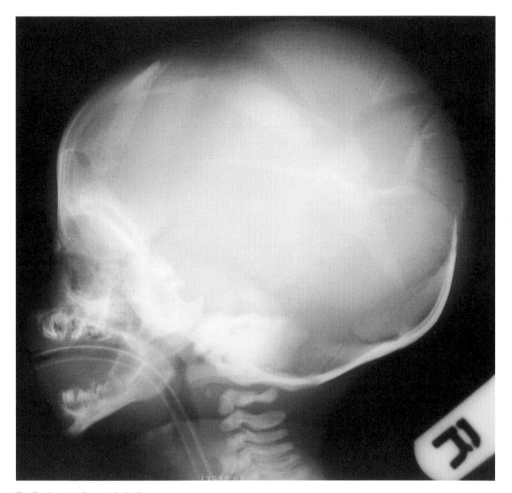

B: Patient 1: Lateral skull

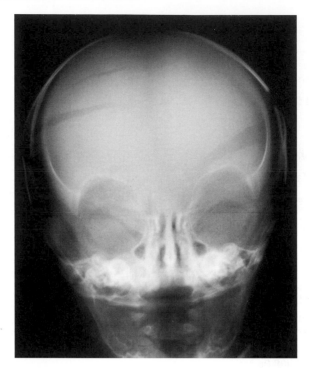

C: Patient 2: AP skull

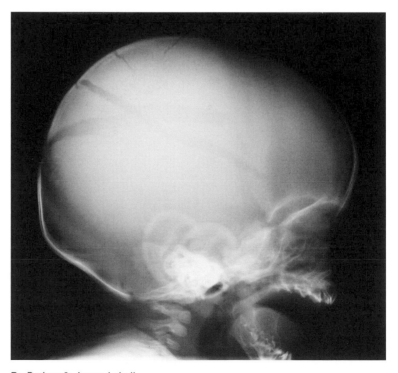

D: Patient 2: Lateral skull

2.6 STELLATE SKULL FRACTURE

Age of fracture:	Less than 10 days (soft tissue swelling on CT)
Degree of force:	Severe (complex fissured (branching) fractures, >4 mm wide, cross sutures to involve all bones, elevated fragment illustrated on CT scan)
Mechanism:	Fall plus gravity onto hard surface/object
Height of fall:	>6 feet
Prevalence in abuse:	Common (7%–30%)
Specificity for abuse:	High (in the absence of an acceptable history)

➡ Fissured, branching or stellate fractures are more likely to occur following an impact against an object with a relatively small surface area, rather than a flat, large surface area.

➡ The history given by this infant's father was of swinging her by her feet so that her head impacted with a glancing blow against the metal arm of a sofa. A square fragment of the outer table was displaced under the scalp to a position more over the vertex.

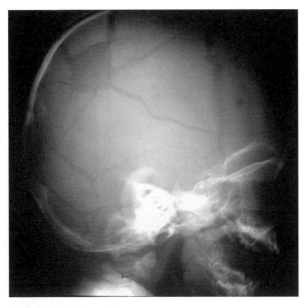

A: Lateral skull

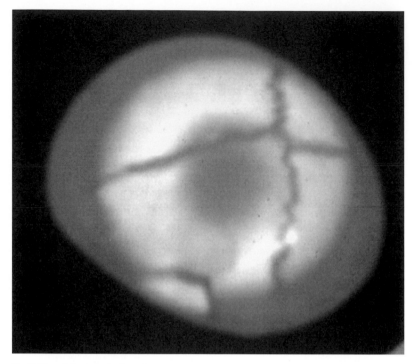

B: CT head (bony windows)

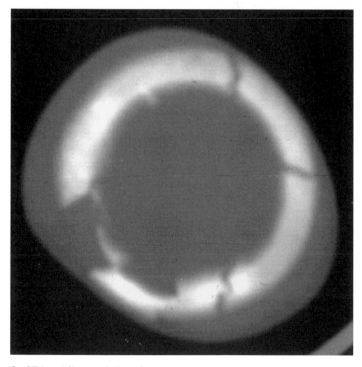

C: CT head (bony windows)

2.7 FISSURED (BRANCHING) OCCIPITAL FRACTURE

Age of fracture:	Uncertain (soft tissue swelling not apparent)
Degree of force:	Severe (complex fissured (branching) fracture, non parietal, >4 mm wide)
Mechanism:	Fall plus gravity onto hard surface/object
Height of fall:	>6 feet
Prevalence in abuse:	Common (7%–30%)
Specificity for abuse:	High (in the absence of an acceptable history)

➡ Note the presence of four wormian (intrasutural) bones (asterisks).
➡ Up to ten wormian bones is considered to be within normal limits.

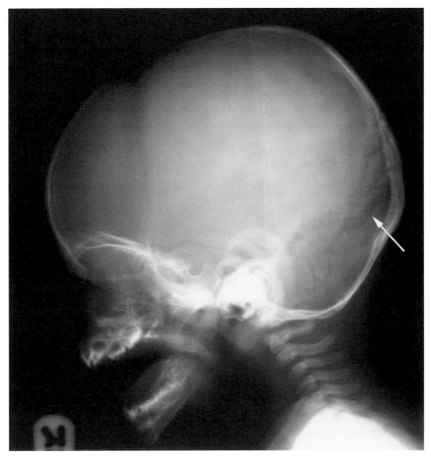

A: Lateral skull

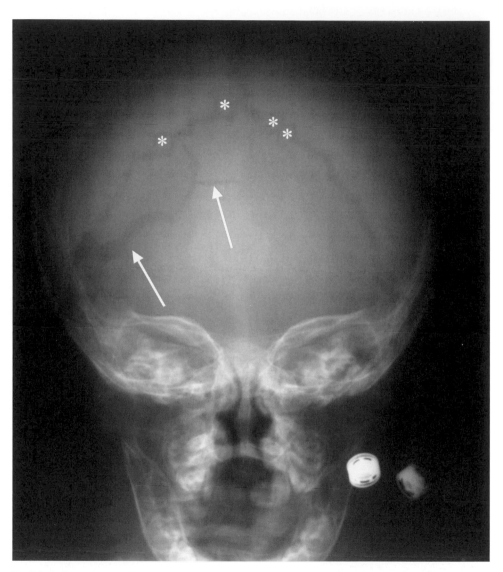

B: AP skull

2.8 SKULL FRACTURES WITH WIDENED SUTURES

Age of fracture:	Uncertain (soft tissue swelling not apparent)
Degree of force:	Severe (associated raised intracranial pressure)
Mechanism:	Fall plus gravity onto hard surface/object
Height of fall:	>6 feet
Prevalence in abuse:	Common (7%–30%)
Specificity for abuse:	High (in the absence of an acceptable history)

➡ Widening of the cranial sutures (arrows) is evidence of raised intracranial pressure, and highly suggestive of intracranial haemorrhage.

➡ In the context of suspected abuse, CT brain should be performed regardless of whether a skull fracture/signs of raised intracranial pressure are evident on the skull radiographs.

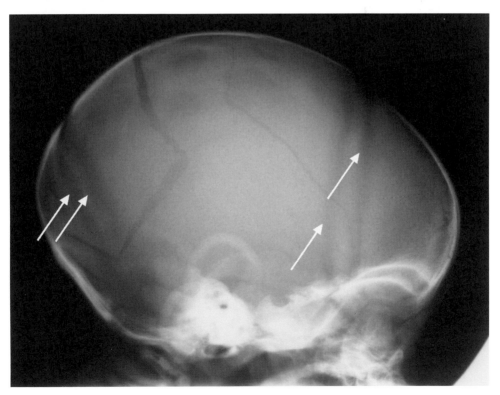

A: Patient 1: Lateral skull

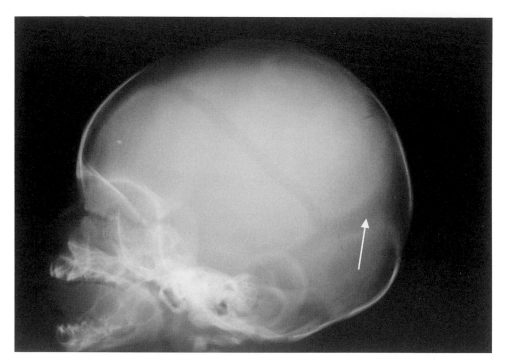

B: Patient 2: Lateral skull

2.9 BIPARIETAL FRACTURES

Age of fracture:	Less than 10 days (soft tissue swelling on CT)
Degree of force:	Severe
Mechanism:	Single midline impact over lambda or a crushing injury
Height of fall:	>6 feet
Prevalence in abuse:	Common (7%–30%)
Specificity for abuse:	High (in the absence of an acceptable history)

➥ Notice how the wider (left) fracture is difficult to demonstrate on CT (*see* Plate 2.2).

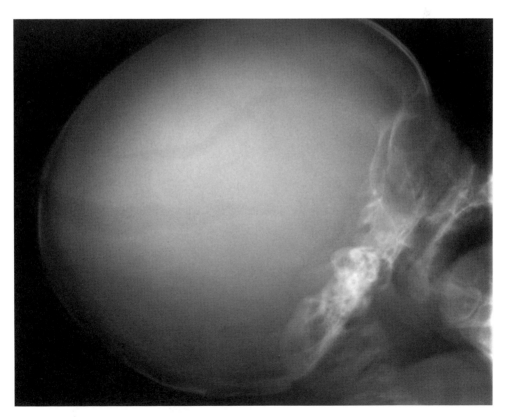

A: Lateral skull

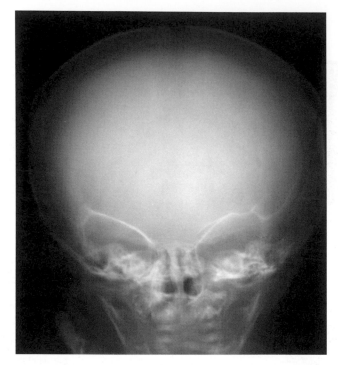

B: AP skull

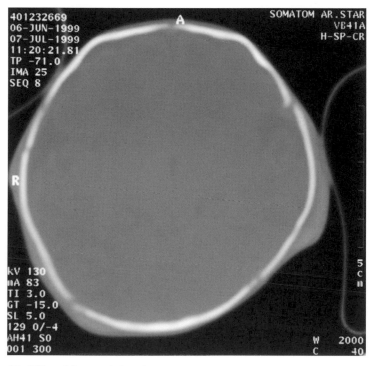

C1: CT head (bony windows)

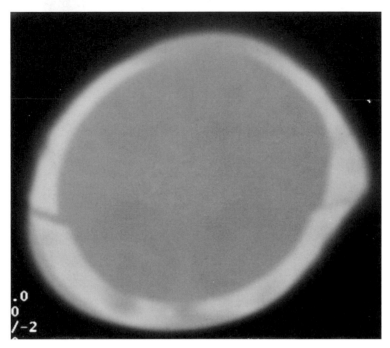

C2: CT head (bony windows)

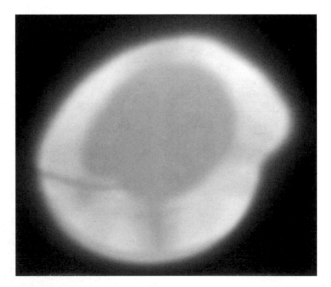

C3: CT head (bony windows)

2.10 3D CT RECONSTRUCTION OF SKULL FRACTURES

Age of fracture:	Uncertain (soft tissue swelling not apparent)
Degree of force:	Severe (complex fracture involving both parietal bones and right side of occiput)
Mechanism:	Fall plus gravity
Height of fall:	>6 feet
Prevalence in abuse:	Common (7%–30%)
Specificity for abuse:	High (in the absence of an acceptable history)

➡ 3D CT reconstruction is helpful to determine the precise course of complex fractures.

➡ Note the single wormian bone in the right lambdoid suture (asterisk).

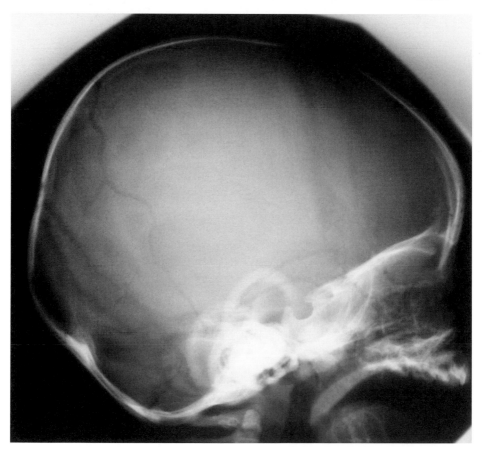

A: Lateral skull

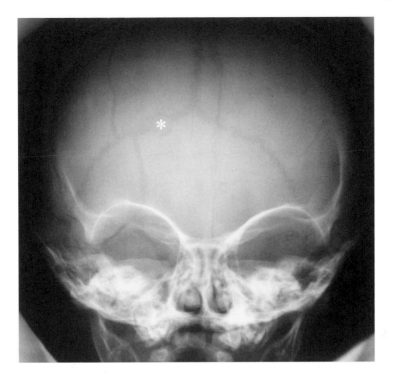

B: AP skull

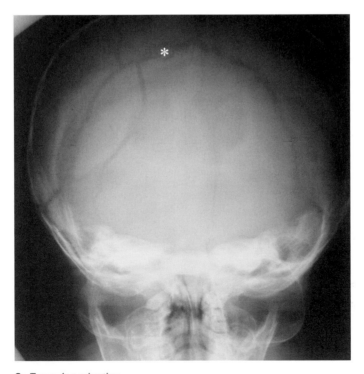

C: Towne's projection

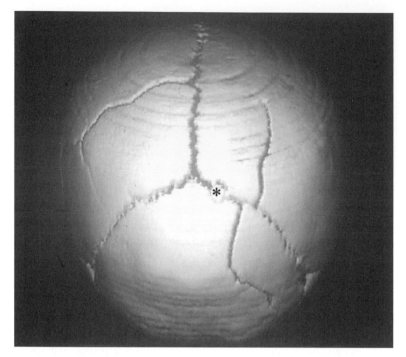

D: 3D CT reconstruction (posterior view)

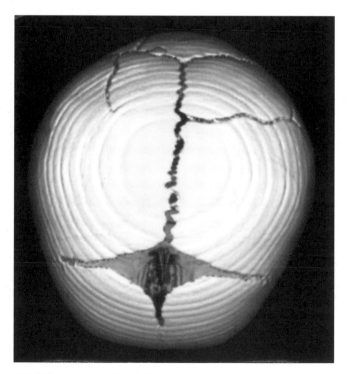

D: 3D CT reconstruction (anterior view)

2.11 PARIETAL FRACTURE + METOPIC SUTURE + INCA BONES

Age of fracture:	Less than 10 days (soft tissue swelling on CT)
Degree of force:	Moderate (simple fracture, <4 mm wide)
Mechanism:	Simple/domestic fall
Height of fall:	3.5 to 5 feet
Prevalence in abuse:	Common (7%–30%)
Specificity for abuse:	Low (commonest fracture in both accidental injury and physical abuse)

➡ On the AP projection, note two normal variants:
  ▪ midline metopic suture (arrow)
  ▪ inca bones (asterisks).

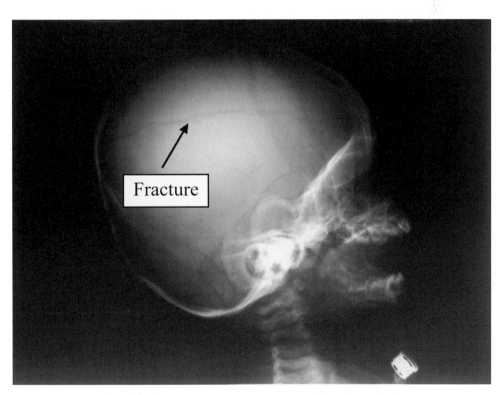

A: Lateral skull

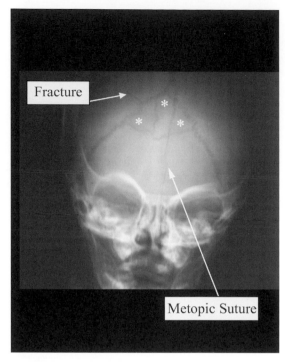

B: AP skull

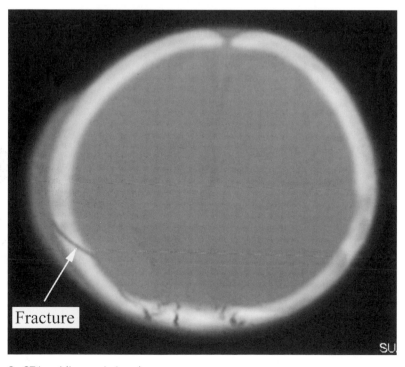

C: CT head (bony windows)

CHAPTER 3

Ribs

In infants, one or more rib fractures may be identified as an incidental finding on a chest radiograph. In this situation they are extremely uncommon. They are more commonly identified on a skeletal survey performed for suspected physical abuse. Although resulting in pain to the infant they are clinically silent in that they are not usually associated with overlying swelling or bruising and are usually not apparent on clinical examination of the infant. Sometimes carers report a sensation of clicking or crackling (crepitus) on holding the chest of the infant, as the broken ends grate over each other in the first few days after the fractures have occurred. Occasionally, fingertip bruising may be seen on the infant's chest, but not overlying the position of the fractures; the fractures occur at some distance from the position of the fingertip force, at the point of maximum bending deformity of the ribs. The usual lack of overlying swelling relates to the fact that rib fractures are rarely displaced because of the relative rigidity of the rib cage and strong intercostal muscles. Displaced rib fractures do result in chest wall swelling and may also be associated with a haemothorax.

POSITION AND MECHANISMS OF CAUSATION

Rib fractures may be identified anywhere along the length of the ribs. They most commonly result from squeezing, compressive forces applied to the chest. This is the typical mechanism when groups or runs of fractures are seen one above the other. The fractures result from significant bending of the ribs during the course of squeezing and occur at the site of maximum distortion of the rib cage. This means that they tend to occur at right angles to the major direction of the squeezing force. In other words a front-to-back compression will result in fractures at the sides of the chest in the mid-axillary lines toward the anterior ends of the ribs.

Posterior rib fractures adjacent to the spine may be caused by side-to-side compression, with the posterior ends being levered over the transverse processes of the spine, which act as the pivots or fulcrums. An alternative mechanism for causing posterior rib fractures has been postulated, whereby the fingertips of adult hands applied around the chest at the back of the infant, force the spine forwards again resulting in a similar levering action over the transverse processes of the spine.

Rarely an isolated rib fracture may have an alternative mechanism of causation; namely a localised direct impact at the site of the fracture. A bruise from the impact would be more likely following this mechanism.

Anterior or costochondral junction fractures may be the result of specific squeezing forces with adult hands around the chest, and the thumbs at the front of the chest overly the costochondral junctions and supply the requisite forces. Alternatively these fractures may result from a direct impact or blow to the epigastrium. This is more commonly the mechanism in the older toddler age group. This mechanism often results in additional intra-abdominal injury such as laceration of the liver, transection of the pancreas or rupture of a hollow viscus, typically the duodenum. There is high morbidity and mortality associated with intra-abdominal injury.

DEFORMITY

It is unusual for rib fractures to show significant displacement because of the rigid configuration of the chest wall and strong intercostal muscles. Occasionally a crushing force may result in several fractures along the length of an individual rib and of adjacent ribs, resulting in a 'flail chest' with associated respiratory distress. In this situation the chest wall is no longer rigid and displacement of the ribs may occur. Displaced rib fractures may result in a pneumothorax, pneumomediastinum or surgical emphysema in the soft tissues and pleural fluid (haemothorax) may be visible on the chest radiograph. Displaced rib fractures may also result in overlying soft tissue swelling.

RIB FRACTURE HEALING

The fracture healing process and dating are exactly as indicated for diaphyseal fractures. There is much less variability in the appearance of healing because of the splinting of the chest wall and the typically undisplaced nature of rib fractures.

— Rib fractures in the early phase may be invisible until the development of soft callus. There are several reasons for failing to identify acute rib fractures.
  - The ribs are superimposed on the lung fields with the complex vascular and bronchial markings masking the fracture lines.
  - The fronts of the ribs are superimposed on the posterior arcs of the ribs.
  - The ribs form continuous curves and the fracture lines can only be seen if they are in the same plane as the X-ray beam. The standard anteroposterior projection therefore cannot demonstrate acute fractures towards the sides of the infant. For this reason, a skeletal survey being undertaken for suspected abuse should include two additional (left and right) oblique views of the chest. Radionuclide scans may also identify unsuspected rib fractures or a delayed chest radiograph (after about two weeks) may demonstrate the presence of callus.
  - Specimen radiographs of the ribs after post-mortem examination may well identify evidence of more fractures, not apparent on the initial study.
— Costochondral junction fractures behave differently from other rib fractures (shaft fractures). They represent the metaphysis of the rib and the healing process is analogous to healing metaphyseal fractures. The fracture line gradually becomes indistinct and consolidates over the course of a few weeks.

EFFECT OF RIB FRACTURES

— Pain, as soon as the fractures occur, resulting in the demonstration of pain, e.g., excessive crying.
— Ongoing pain for several days following the fractures, on any direct handling of the chest, resulting in further demonstration of pain. This may not be localised by the regular carers and may be put down to other childhood ailments such as colic, teething or earache.
— Rapid, shallow breathing by the infant for a few days in an attempt to reduce the painful effect of the rib fractures. The carers may not note this.
— Fingertip bruising (but typically no bruising or swelling overlies the fractures).

DIFFERENTIAL DIAGNOSIS

— Some expanding lytic areas may be seen in a rare enchondroma or fibrous dysplasia or Langerhans' cell histiocytoma and be mistaken for healing fractures.

— Rib fractures may occur following normal handling or physiotherapy in infants with underlying metabolic bone disease, renal disease or osteopathy of prematurity, or those with severe forms of osteogenesis imperfecta (Type III).

— More commonly, rib fractures are mistakenly diagnosed as a result of misinterpretation of normal radiographic findings. These include an apparent expansion of the posterior ends of some ribs from the superimposition of the posterior ends of the ribs and the transverse processes of the spine. Also, on oblique views of the chest, the rounded sternal centres superimposed on the ribs may be mistaken for healing rib fractures.

— Rib fractures occur extremely rarely as a result of birth trauma. They have been described following a difficult delivery with shoulder dystocia in large infants of more than four kilograms. They may also occur as a result of a difficult and traumatic forceps delivery.

— Cardiac resuscitation results in rib fractures extremely rarely. Several series have demonstrated that this is the case whether lay people or healthcare professionals performed the resuscitation. On the few occasions that rib fractures have been reported they have occurred in the mid-axillary line, affecting the 7th–9th ribs.

3.1 POSTERIOR RIB FRACTURES: HEALING (2–4 WEEKS)

Age of fractures: Solid arrows: about 2 weeks (early callus)

Degree of force: Significant

Mechanism: Squeezing/compressive side-to-side force

Prevalence in abuse: Probably high, but under-reported[68]

Specificity for abuse: High

➥ Note the fracture of the left 10th rib posteriorly (dashed arrow). This fracture is approximately 4 weeks of age (more mature callus, fracture line still visible).

➥ Isolated rib fractures may occur from blunt trauma in which case there may be an overlying bruise.

➥ *See* Plates 3.2 and 3.3.

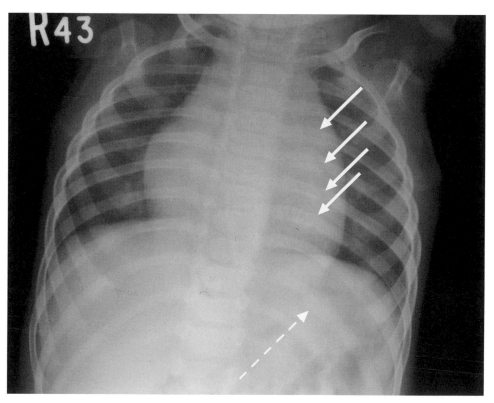

AP chest

3.2 POSTERIOR RIB FRACTURES: HEALING (4–6 WEEKS)

Age of fractures: 4–6 weeks (mature callus, visible fracture line)

Degree of force: Significant

Mechanism: Squeezing/compressive side-to-side force

Prevalence in abuse: Probably high, but under-reported[68]

Specificity for abuse: High

➥ This is the same child as that shown in Plates 3.1 and 3.3. This radiograph
  was performed 18 days after initial presentation.
➥ Notice how, by the time of the delayed radiograph, callus formation
  emphasises the presence of rib fractures. It is for this reason that chest
  radiographs performed 10–14 days after initial presentation have been
  advocated for the *routine investigation* of suspected abuse in infants and
  children less than 2 years.
➥ *See* Plates 3.1 and 3.3.

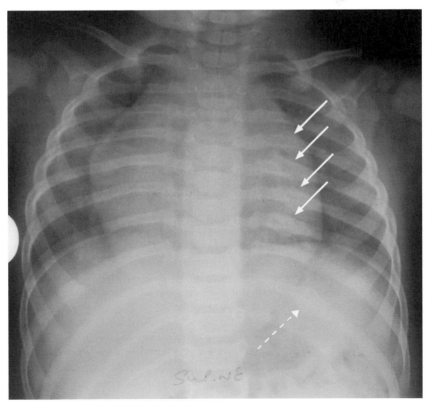

AP chest

3.3 POSTERIOR RIB FRACTURES: HEALING (9–11 WEEKS)

Age of fractures:	Left: 8 weeks + (mature callus, no visible fracture line) Right: 11 weeks + (more mature callus, some remodelling)
Degree of force:	Significant
Mechanism:	Squeezing/compressive side-to-side force
Prevalence in abuse:	Probably high, but under-reported[68]
Specificity for abuse:	High

➥ This is the same child as that shown in Plates 3.1 and 3.2. This radiograph was performed 53 days after initial presentation.
➥ Notice the lack of modelling deformity of the left 5th to 7th ribs.
➥ Right-sided healing rib fractures are now visible. These are not detectable on the earlier radiographs (even with hindsight).
➥ *Research question: How delayed should 'delayed' radiographs be?*
➥ *See* Plates 3.1 and 3.2

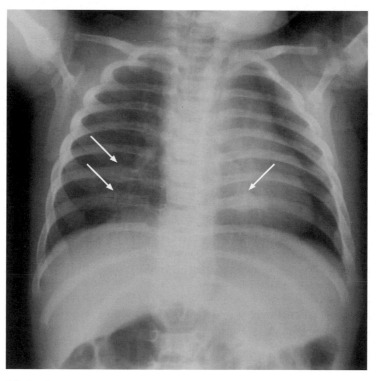

AP chest

3.4 LATERAL RIB FRACTURES: ACUTE (<7 DAYS)

Age of fractures: <7 days (no callus, visible fracture lines)

Degree of force: Significant

Mechanism: Squeezing/compressive front-to-back force

Prevalence in abuse: Probably high, but under-reported[68]

Specificity for abuse: High

➥ Notice displaced fracture ends.
➥ Notice left pleural fluid (haemothorax) and swelling of left chest wall.
➥ Cardiopulmonary resuscitation is an uncommon cause of mid-axillary line fractures of the 7th to 9th ribs.
➥ The acute fractures in the mid-axillary line are visible because of their displacement. Non-displaced acute fractures in this position may not have been visible on this single projection.
➥ *See* Plates 3.5 and 3.6.

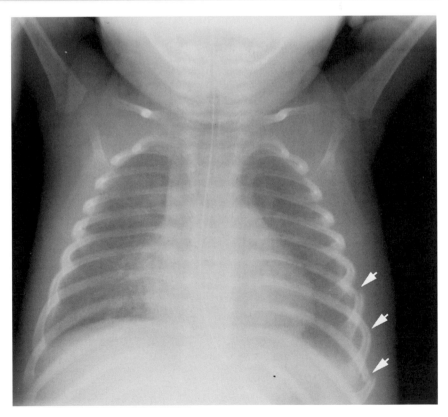

AP chest

3.5 MULTIPLE RIB FRACTURES: HEALING (2–3 WEEKS)

Age of fractures: 2–3 weeks + (early callus, visible fracture lines)

Degree of force: Significant

Mechanism: Squeezing/compressive side-to-side and front-to-back forces

Prevalence in abuse: Probably high, but under-reported[68]

Specificity for abuse: High

→ This is the same child as that shown in Plates 3.4 and 3.6. This radiograph was performed 14 days after initial presentation.
→ Multiple left and right, anterior, lateral and posterior fractures are demonstrated (arrows point to some – not all – fractures).
→ *See* Plates 3.4 and 3.6.

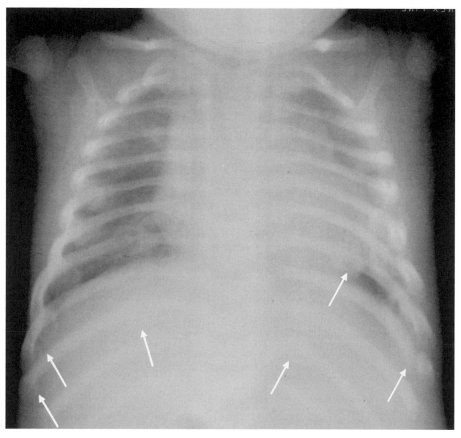

AP chest

3.6 RIB FRACTURES: HEALING (6–7 WEEKS)

Age of fractures:	6 weeks + (mature callus, no visible fracture line)
Degree of force:	Significant
Mechanism:	Squeezing/compressive side-to-side and front-to-back forces
Prevalence in abuse:	Probably high, but under-reported[68]
Specificity for abuse:	High

➥ This is the same child as that shown in Plates 3.4 and 3.5. This radiograph was performed 43 days after initial presentation.
➥ Many of the posterior rib fractures are beginning to remodel.
➥ Significant callus formation of the left lateral rib fractures is related to the degree of displacement of the original rib fractures.
➥ Note also the fracture of the right clavicle.
➥ *See* Plates 3.4 and 3.5.

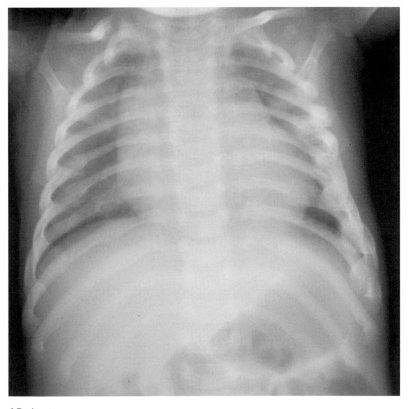

AP chest

3.7 RIB FRACTURES: IN TWIN OF INDEX CASE

Age of fractures: Acute and healing

Degree of force: Significant

Mechanism: Squeezing/compressive side-to-side and front-to-
                      back forces

Prevalence in abuse: Probably high, but under-reported[68]

Specificity for abuse: High

➥ This is the twin of the child shown in Plates 3.4–3.6. These radiographs
  were performed on day of admission (A) and 36 days later (B).
➥ When abuse is diagnosed in one child, it is important to perform a skeletal
  survey on any siblings under two years of age (some say under three
  years of age).
➥ *Research question: Up to what age should we routinely investigate
  siblings of index cases?*

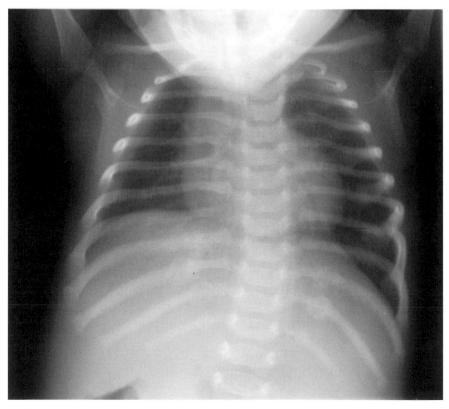

A: AP chest

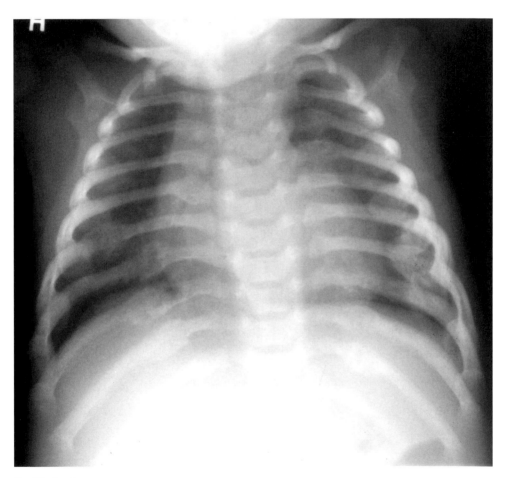

B: AP chest

3.8 RIB FRACTURES: COSTOCHONDRAL

Age of fractures:	Acute, <2 weeks (fracture line still clearly visible)
Degree of force:	Significant
Mechanism:	Squeezing over costochondral junction or Direct blow to epigastrium
Prevalence in abuse:	Uncommon
Specificity for abuse:	High

➡ Costochondral junction fractures are analogous to long bone CMLs and heal in the same way (gradual resolution of fracture line with insignificant callus formation).
➡ Costochondral junction fractures are often associated with intra-abdominal injury as in this case – *see* Plate 7.6 (pancreatic laceration with pseudocyst formation).

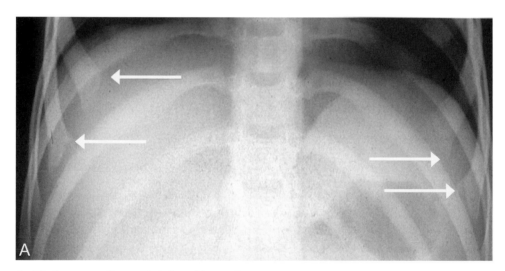

A: AP chest, coned/magnified view of lower ribs

3.9 RIB FRACTURES: DETECTED ON BONE SCAN

Age of fractures:	Isotope bone scans cannot be used to date fractures That they are visible on the scan and not on the radiograph implies they are either acute (<7 days) or old (>12 weeks)
Degree of force:	Significant
Mechanism:	Squeezing/compressive side-to-side force
Prevalence in abuse:	Probably high, but under-reported[68]
Specificity for abuse:	High

➡ High quality Technetium 99 isotope bone scans play a complementary role to the skeletal survey in investigating suspected physical abuse. They are not routinely performed in all centres.

➡ *Research question: What is the effectiveness/cost effectiveness of routine isotope bone scans in addition to (or instead of) skeletal surveys for the investigation of suspected abuse?*

➡ Posterior rib fractures seen on bone scan (A) are present but not readily identified on the radiograph (B).

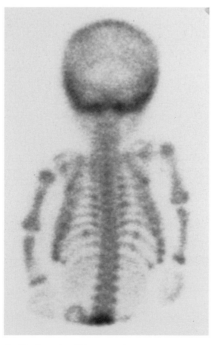

A: Technetium[99] isotope bone scan

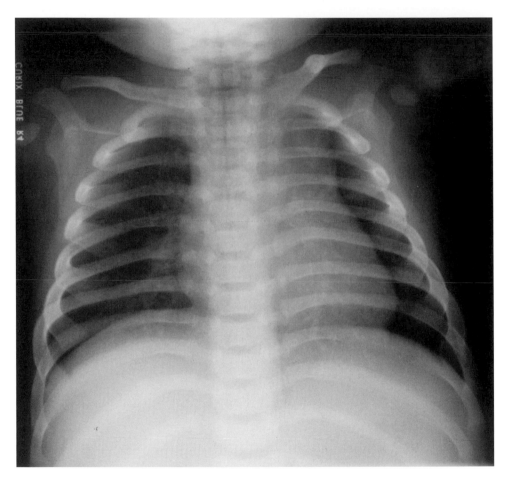

B: AP chest

3.10 RIB FRACTURES: DETECTED ON BONE SCAN

Age of fracture:	Isotope bone scans cannot be used to date fractures
Degree of force:	Significant
Mechanism:	Squeezing/compressive side-to-side force
Prevalence in abuse:	Probably high, but under-reported[68]
Specificity for abuse:	High

- ➡ The rib fractures seen as increased tracer uptake (hotspots) on the bone scan are not demonstrable on the radiograph.
- ➡ Note the fracture of the right clavicle (arrows).
- ➡ Normal increased tracer uptake at the growth plates and skull vault obscures CMLs and skull fractures, therefore bone scans MUST be supplemented with radiographs when abuse is suspected.

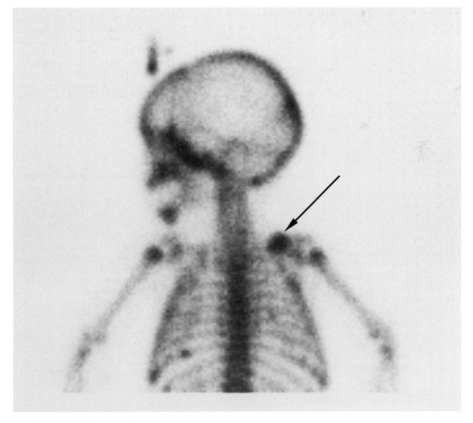

A: Technetium[99] isotope bone scan

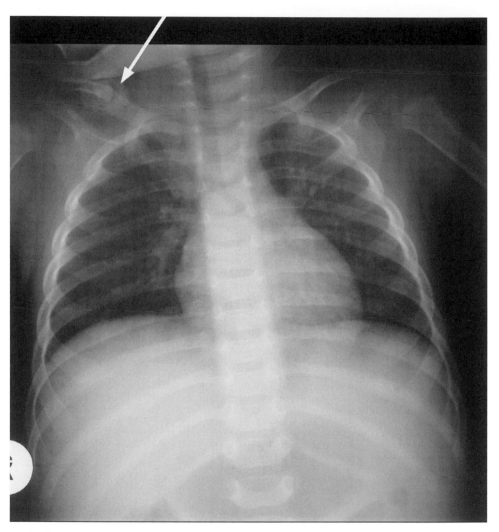

B: AP Chest

3.11 RIB FRACTURES: NOT DETECTED ON BONE SCAN

Age of fractures:	Isotope bone scans cannot be used to date fractures
	Age as assessed from chest radiograph: 6 weeks +
Degree of force:	Significant
Mechanism:	Squeezing/compressive side-to-side and front-to-back forces
Prevalence in abuse:	Probably high, but under-reported[68]
Specificity for abuse:	High

⇢ Poor quality isotope bone scan (compare degree of tracer uptake to that in Plates 3.9 and 3.10).
⇢ The healing rib fractures demonstrated on the radiograph are not identified on the bone scan.
⇢ Notice the increased radioisotope uptake at the site of the right distal humeral fracture.

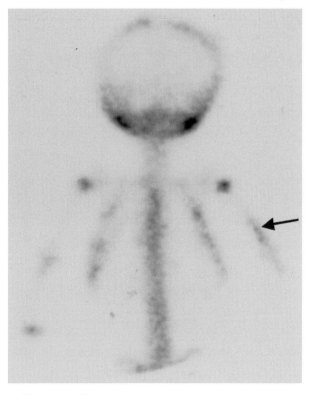

A: Technetium[99] isotope bone scan

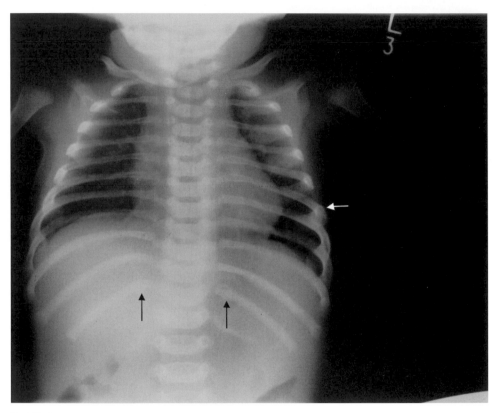

B: AP chest

3.12 RIB FRACTURES: ADVANTAGE OF FAXITRON IMAGES

➥ Faxitron images are post-mortem specimen radiographs.
➥ They involve significantly higher radiation exposure than standard radiographs, for example at our institution, parameters for an infant are as follows:
  ▶ chest radiograph: mAs = 2, Kv = 60
  ▶ faxitron: mAs = 25, Kv = 65.
➥ Faxitron images allow more precise demonstration and dating of rib fractures.

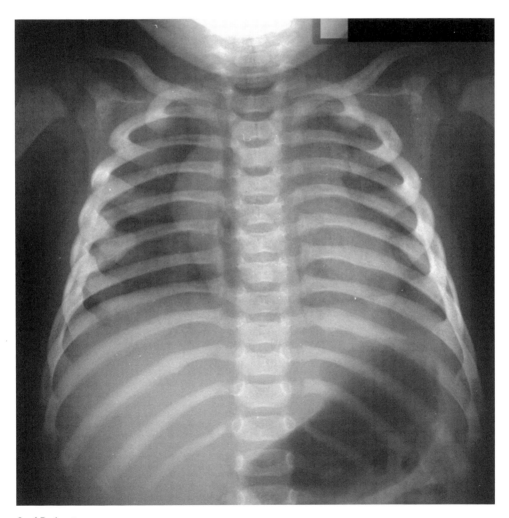

A: AP chest

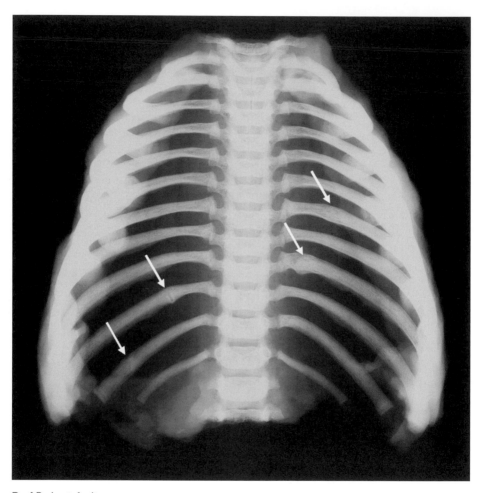

B: AP chest, faxitron

3.13 RIB FRACTURES: ADVANTAGE OF FAXITRON IMAGES

➡ Notice the improved demonstration of the healing fractures of the left posterior 5th and 7th ribs and left 8th rib in the mid-axillary line on the faxitron image (broken arrows).

➡ Also note the demonstration of the previously unidentified fracture of the right 7th costochondral junction (solid arrow).

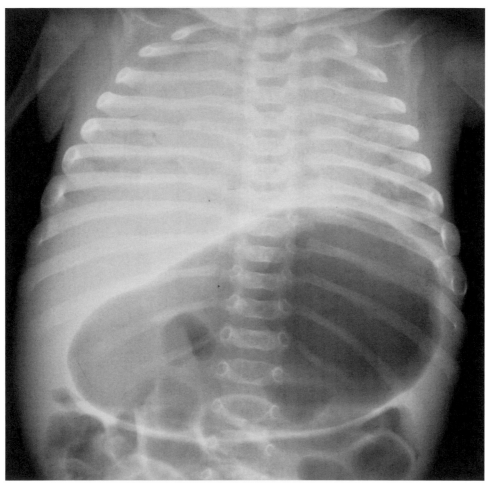

A: AP chest

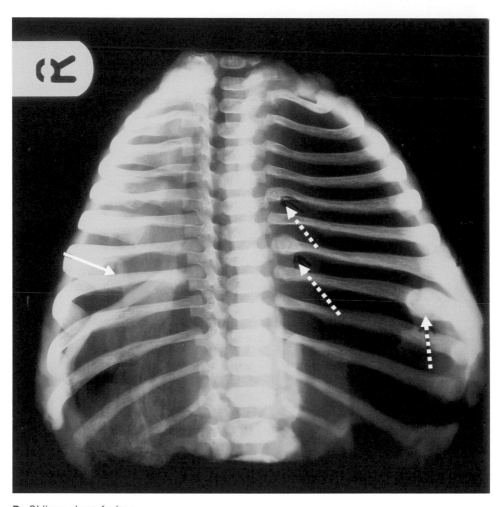

B: Oblique chest, faxitron

3.14 RIB FRACTURES: HISTOPATHOLOGY

➥ Post-mortem histopathology complements skeletal surveys and faxitron images in the investigation of sudden unexpected death in infancy.

➥ Gross histology (A) is better at detecting acute rib fractures (blood clot) than radiography (B).

➥ Radiography is advantageous in detecting healing fractures as it guides the pathologist as to the specific rib/site from which to prepare the histology slides (C & D).

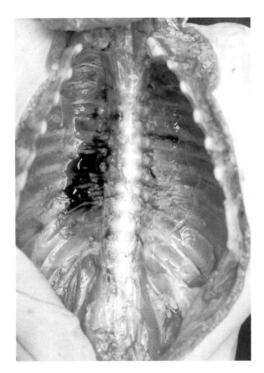

A: Gross anatomy

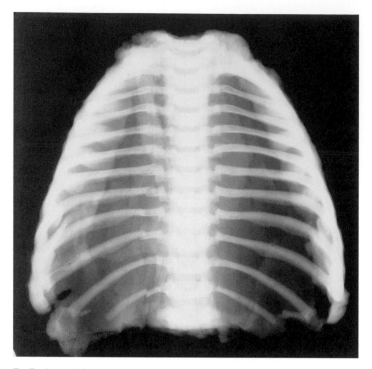

B: Faxitron, AP chest

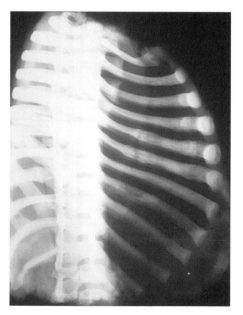

C: Faxitron, right oblique

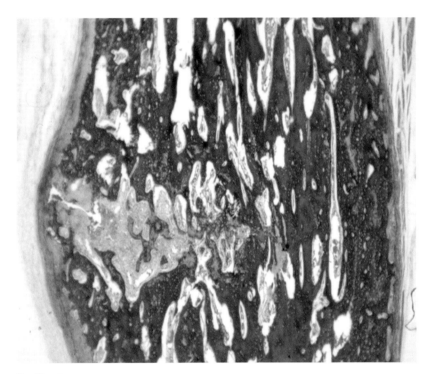

D: Histology

CHAPTER 4

Flat bones and spine

4.1 SHOULDER GIRDLE: ACROMION (ACUTE)

Age of fracture: Acute (no callus formation, sharp fracture margins)

Degree of force: Significant

Mechanism: Rotation/traction applied to shoulder/upper limb
                      Indirect forces generated during shaking

Prevalence in abuse: Rare

Specificity for abuse: High

➥ The acromion is the commonest site for scapula fractures (solid arrows).
➥ In this patient, notice the multiple rib fractures of varying age
  (arrowheads), and the fractures of the distal radial shaft and ulna
  metaphysis (broken arrows).

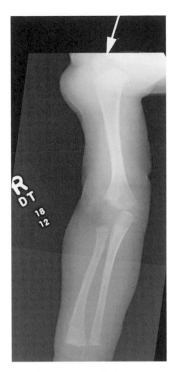

A: AP right upper limb

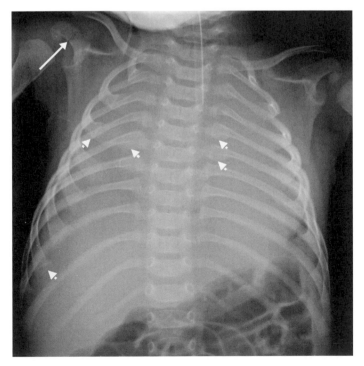

B: AP chest

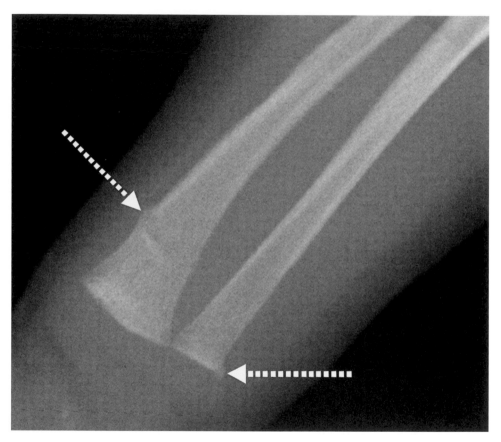

C: AP right forearm (magnified)

4.2 SHOULDER GIRDLE: ACROMION (HEALING)

Age of fracture:	2–4 weeks (callus formation, visible fracture line with irregular margins)
Degree of force:	Significant
Mechanism:	Rotation/traction applied to shoulder/upper limb Indirect forces generated during shaking
Prevalence in abuse:	Rare
Specificity for abuse:	High

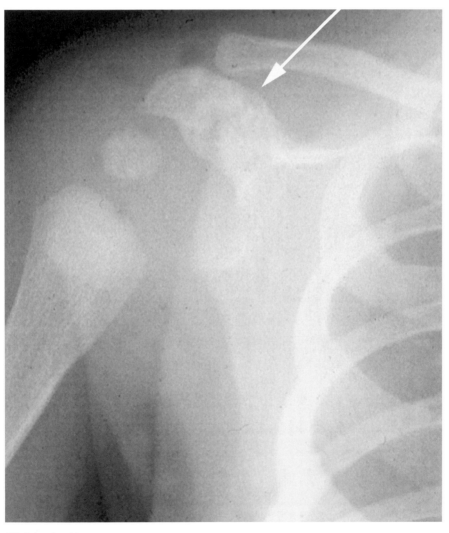

AP right shoulder

4.3 SHOULDER GIRDLE: LATERAL END OF CLAVICLE

Age of fracture:	2–4 weeks (some callus formation, fracture line visible)
Degree of force:	Significant
Mechanism:	Uncertain
Prevalence in abuse:	Rare
Specificity for abuse:	High

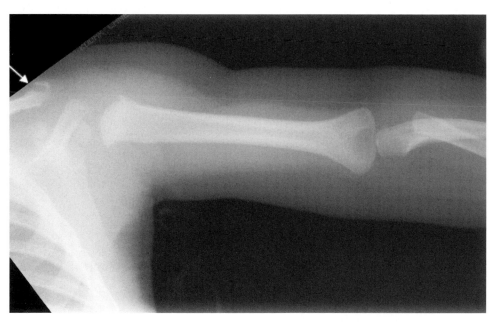

AP left shoulder

4.4 SHOULDER GIRDLE: BODY OF SCAPULA

Age of fracture: 2–4 weeks (surrounding sclerosis and relatively
                       indistinct fracture margins are signs of healing)

Degree of force: Significant

Mechanism: Uncertain (possibly a direct blow)

Prevalence in abuse: Rare[23]

Specificity for abuse: High

➡ Notice improved visualisation on the post-mortem faxitron radiograph (B).

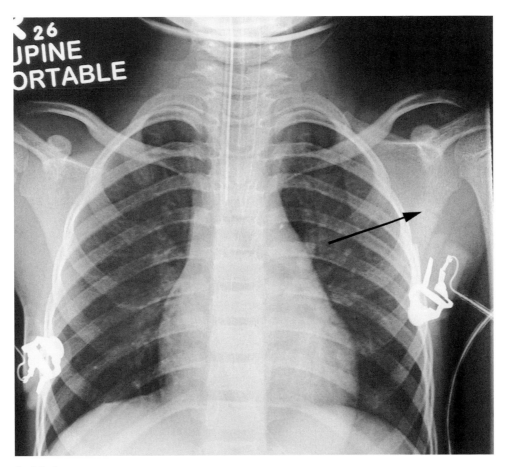

A: AP chest

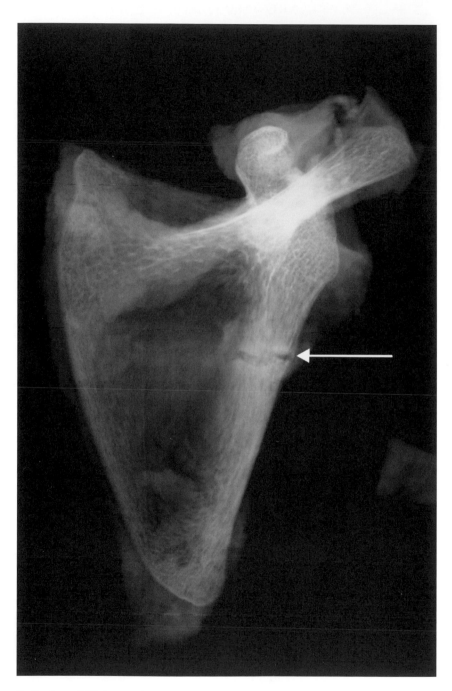

B: Faxitron, AP left scapula

4.5 SPINE

Age of fracture:	These fractures are not possible to date. There is no healing response but rather a gradual return to normal vertebral body height
Degree of force:	Significant
Mechanism:	Hyperflexion/axial loading with or without a rotational component (diffuse loss of height)
Prevalence in abuse:	Rare (<3%)
Specificity for abuse:	High

➡ This child was thrown out of a caravan door onto concrete, by the mother's partner, and landed on his head.

➡ Although vertebral fractures may occur at any site, they are commonest at the thoracolumbar junction.

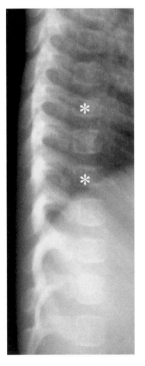

Lateral thoracic spine

4.6 SPINE

Age of fracture:	These fractures are not possible to date. There is no healing response but rather a gradual return to normal vertebral body height
Degree of force:	Significant
Mechanism:	Hyperflexion (mainly anterior loss of height)
Prevalence in abuse:	Rare (<3%)
Specificity for abuse:	High

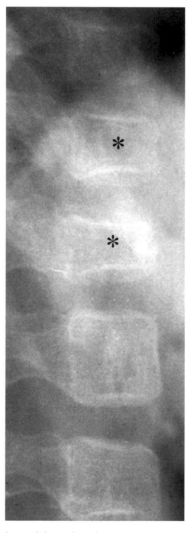

Lateral thoracic spine

4.7 SPINE

Age of fracture:	These fractures are not possible to date. There is no healing response but rather a gradual return to normal vertebral body height
Degree of force:	Significant
Mechanism:	Hyperflexion (mainly anterior loss of height)
Prevalence in abuse:	Rare (<3%)
Specificity for abuse:	High

➡ Injury may result in fracture of multiple vertebrae, or (as in this case) involve only a single vertebral body.

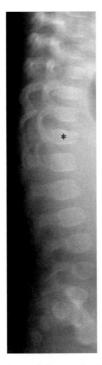

Lateral thoracolumbar
spine

4.8 PELVIS: FRACTURE OF SUPERIOR PUBIC RAMUS

Age of fracture: 5–7 weeks (callus with visible fracture line)

Degree of force: Significant

Mechanism: Uncertain (possibly direct impact)

Prevalence in abuse: Rare (<1%)

Specificity for abuse: High

➠ Some infants demonstrate normal synchondroses (*see* Plate 8.3) in this position because of development from two ossification centres. This represents a normal variant that needs differentiation. This case can be seen to be a fracture because of the development of callus. If there is doubt about the finding then delayed radiographs (10–14 days) should demonstrate no change in the case of a normal variant, but the development of callus with a fracture.

➠ Note absence of ossification of the proximal femoral epiphyses indicating the young age of this infant.

➠ These fractures may be seen in association with sexual abuse as in the child who also had a ruptured rectum (*see* Plate 7.9).

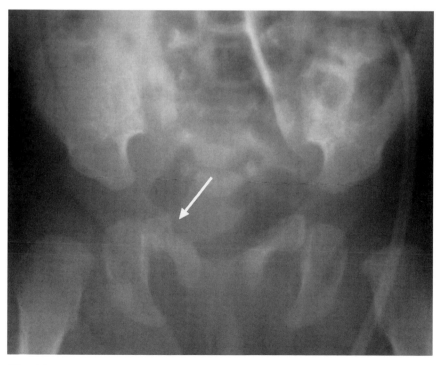

AP pelvis

CHAPTER 5

Diaphyseal fractures

A diaphyseal or shaft fracture affects a long bone of one of the limbs and is often the presenting skeletal injury in infants who have been the subject of physical abuse. The pain, deformity and swelling often associated with a diaphyseal fracture, together with the immobility (pseudo-paralysis) of the limb, are usually readily apparent to the carers of the injured infant.

PATTERNS AND MECHANISMS OF CAUSATION OF DIAPHYSEAL FRACTURES

Different patterns of diaphyseal fractures are recognised and each indicates the major mechanism of causation of an individual fracture.

— A transverse fracture, at right angles to the axis of the long bone, may be caused by one of two mechanisms.
  - Firstly, it may be the result of a direct impact of a hard object at the site of the fracture. This may either be the result of the infant being forcefully moved so as to come into contact with a hard object, for example by being swung, thrown or dropped from a height; or by a hard moving object coming into contact with the immobile infant, if used as an implement or thrown or falling from a height.
  - Secondly, a transverse fracture may result from an applied levering force, with the pivot or fulcrum being at the site of the fracture. If the fracture is the result of a levering force it is more likely to be associated with some angulation at the site of the fracture.
— Spiral and oblique fractures are considered to be the same and the result of the same mechanisms. On one radiographic projection the fracture line may appear to be oblique, passing in a straight line at an angle across the shaft of the bone, and in another projection the same fracture has a twisting, spiral appearance. A spiral fracture is the result of a twisting (torsional) force applied to the limb, either distal to (below) the site of the fracture, or proximal to (above) the site of the fracture. For example a spiral fracture of the humerus may be the result of a rapid gripping twisting force applied around the region of the elbow and forearm, or the result of the infant's body twisting during the course of being swung by one arm.
— Other types of fractures are less common in infancy, although more common in older active children following accidents. These would include:
  - a torus fracture with the break involving only one side of the shaft
  - a greenstick fracture, also with a break on one side but with a component extending along the axis of the long bone
  - a buckle fracture with a bending circumferentially around the shaft, but with no clear fracture line, and
  - a bowing fracture due to multiple micro-fractures causing the length of the shaft to bend.

These fractures are occasionally seen in infants, but their mechanisms of causation are often not clear.

In infants, any fracture needs a clear account of the causative incident and may be the result of accidental or non-accidental trauma. Bruising may or may not be associated with a diaphyseal fracture and relates to the surface area over which a force has been applied. For example a direct impact by a small object would be more likely to result in bruising than a force exerted by a relatively larger gripping adult hand.

DEFORMITY

This is the result of varying combinations of:
— soft tissue processes:
  • deep swelling from bleeding from the broken ends of the bone
  • superficial oedema.
— bone deformity at the site of the fracture:
  • separation
  • angulation
  • overlap.

SOFT TISSUE CHANGES ASSOCIATED WITH DIAPHYSEAL FRACTURES

Several factors in relation to diaphyseal fractures will determine the extent of the associated soft tissue change and deformity and also influence the appearances of the healing process.
— The fracture may be undisplaced, appearing as a fine hairline fracture or crack fracture. In this case there would be minimal soft tissue swelling and only a small amount of periosteal new bone formation as evidence of healing, with no, or minimal callus formation. In this situation there may be no soft tissue change visible radiographically and no signs on clinical examination. There would however be the symptoms associated with a fracture – pain on handling the limb and loss of movement of the injured limb (pseudo-paralysis). In a toddler or an infant beginning to stand there would also be inability to weight-bear if the lower limb were fractured. An undisplaced fracture may result in delayed presentation.
— Alternatively there may be significant displacement of the broken ends of the bone with a combination of separation, angulation and overlap. With significant displacement there is rapid development of bleeding from the broken ends of the bone and a deep swelling occurs. In addition, oedema develops in the more superficial tissues; initially, in the first few hours this is localised to around the site of the fracture, but gradually extends up and down the injured limb over the course of a few days. The oedema and deep swelling gradually resolve over the course of about one week, but the whole process of soft tissue swelling may last longer with more major displacement of the fracture.

The radiological appearances are well demonstrated on digital imaging, particularly when soft copy windowing is available. The appearance of the initial deep bleeding is that of an overall increase in the size of the injured area, when compared with the other limb. The radiographic changes due to oedema in the more superficial tissues include the loss of definition of the soft tissue planes and an overall increase in size.

Although the swelling begins immediately after the fracture has occurred, the point at which it is observed or noticed by carers or on clinical examination is variable and depends on several factors.

— The specific type of fracture: each fracture is individual with varying degrees of surface area (greater in a spiral than a transverse fracture), and of separation and deformity.
— The specific bone that has been fractured: for example the swelling from a fractured femur may take longer to be identified because of the chubby soft tissue of the thigh masking the initial swelling process.
— The time of year and therefore the amount of clothing covering the fractured area.
— The carers' levels of awareness.

DEFORMITY ASSOCIATED WITH DIAPHYSEAL FRACTURES

The more angulation and/or overlap there is of the fracture, the more obvious is the deformity of the affected limb. The full extent of the deformity may not be apparent from the standard anteroposterior and lateral radiographs if the maximum displacement is not precisely in line with either of these projections. The deformity almost always occurs immediately at the time of the fracture and is the result of the relative displaced positions of the broken ends of the bone at the site of the fracture. Rarely, further displacement may occur as a result of forceful handling within a few days of the initial fracture, however normal handling in the presence of a diaphyseal fracture, even when the limb has not been immobilised, would not be expected to cause further displacement.

Occasionally, when a diaphyseal fracture has not been adequately immobilised, re-fracturing may occur within the first few weeks of a fracture occurring. Because this is not commonly seen it is thought to be the result of forces beyond the range of normal handling even though the fractured area may be relatively weaker during the healing process.

Although deformity may be a reflection of the relatively greater force required to cause this type of fracture, it is also the result of muscular attachments and powerful muscular spasm. In general the powerful muscles of the thigh result in greater deformity of a fractured femur than for example a fracture of the humerus, and deformity is relatively less pronounced as a result of muscle spasm in the paired bones of the forearm and lower leg.

DIAPHYSEAL FRACTURE HEALING AND DATING

The healing process follows an orderly sequence of both radiological and pathological findings. Both disciplines are able to give estimated age ranges. In general, histopathology can be more refined in dating injuries of less than one week, whereas radiological features give better estimates of older fractures. The radiological findings are inevitably subjective and to some extent accuracy of dating is reflected in the experience of the paediatric radiologist.

— Healing process:
  - 0–7 days.
    The fracture line is crisp with no evidence of any new bone formation. The appearances of the soft tissues may be helpful, particularly in relation to the extent of oedema, depending on whether or not the fracture is displaced. There may be no soft tissue changes in a totally undisplaced fracture. In displaced fractures, oedema extending up and down the limb will take a few days to develop. Minimal oedema, confined to the area of the fracture, may be seen in a recent fracture (within several hours of the fracture occurring), or towards the end of the first seven-day period as the oedema is resolving.

- 7–14 days.
  Early periosteal new bone along the shaft is seen as a faint, thin white line in the region of the fracture. It is the healing response of damage to the periosteum.
- 2–4 weeks.
  The periosteal new bone is clearly defined as a definite white line and extends away from the fracture line along the shaft. In addition, early soft callus becomes visible around the fracture and has a soft, indistinct, fluffy, flocculated appearance. This callus is developing in the framework resulting from the initial deep bleeding from the fractured ends of the bone.
- 4–6 weeks.
  The periosteal reaction is thicker and beginning to consolidate to the adjacent diaphysis. The callus is more consolidated, although still with some flocculation. It appears as a clearly-defined ball of bone around the fracture.
- 6–8 weeks.
  The fracture line becomes very indistinct and disappears during this period. This will only be fully appreciated if the plane of the X-ray beam is the same as that of the fracture. There is more consolidation of both the periosteal new bone, which shows further fusion with the diaphysis and the callus, which is now described as hard callus. The callus appears as a homogeneous focal rounded area of bone around the site of the fracture. There will be early evidence of remodelling, with the edges of callus immediately abutting the diaphysis showing blunting of the angles and beginning to conform to the shape of the shaft.
- 8–12 weeks.
  There is continued remodelling of the hard callus. By twelve weeks there has been almost complete remodelling with only some residual thickening of the shaft. The whole process of remodelling will take longer the greater the degree of bone deformity and separation associated with the original fracture.

This continuous healing process merges from one stage to the next. In general a more precise estimate of the age of a fracture can be given in the earlier stages of fracture healing. The above appearances relate to a moderately displaced (a few millimetres – not hairline) fracture. The appearances of healing will vary depending on several factors (although the ongoing process will remain the same).

— Undisplaced fractures have relatively little deep bleeding at the time of injury and may develop little or no callus. The healing process relates to the periosteal injury and new bone formation.

— Similarly the group of fractures associated with an incomplete break of the outer cortex of the long bone (buckle, greenstick, torus) will show only localised periosteal new bone and some sclerosis as evidence of healing of the fracture within the shaft.

— Displaced fractures (angulated or overlapping) will take much longer for the remodelling process to become complete. Evidence of some residual bone deformity may remain for several years.

— Re-fracture at the same site. The same healing process starts again and is superimposed on the earlier healing process. Estimates of dating of original and re-fractures can only be imprecise but within certain boundaries.

— Active rickets results in failure of ossification of the provisional zone of calcification at the metaphyses. Callus relating to an underlying fracture will also fail to ossify until the rickets is in the healing phase. Active rickets is readily diagnosed radiologically and also from biochemistry.

EXUBERANT CALLUS

The volume of callus around a fracture is not helpful in dating an injury. Excessive or exuberant callus may be seen:
— with a large area of fractured bone (spiral) which is displaced
— with angulated or overlapping fractures
— with failure to immobilise a fracture
— with a bleeding disorder
— in neurological disorders with evidence of insensitivity to pain due to repetitive trauma
— in a rare form of osteogenesis imperfecta also associated with cross-fusion of paired bones (OI type V).

EFFECT OF A DIAPHYSEAL FRACTURE

— Pain, as soon as the fractures occur, resulting in the demonstration of pain, e.g., excessive crying.
— Ongoing pain for about one week following the fracture, on any movement or handling of the injured limb, resulting in further demonstration of pain.
— Inability or unwillingness to move the limb for about one week after the injury, in an attempt to reduce the pain. This results in a pseudo-paralysis of the limb. It will also result in a loss of some motor skills depending on the stage of development. For example an infant may stop crawling or lose the ability to roll.
— Deformity as discussed above.

DIFFERENTIAL DIAGNOSIS

— Accidental trauma. This requires the careful evaluation of the history given in relation to the severity and type of injury sustained. The history given should be consistent over time and between any witnesses of the injury. Evidence of further injury would detract from the diagnosis of accidental trauma.
— Medical/iatrogenic conditions giving rise to osteopenia. Osteopenia may not be apparent radiographically until bone density has reduced by about 30%. It seems that in practice however, fractures do not start occurring spontaneously until there is some evidence of radiographic osteopenia.
  • Most notable would be osteogenesis imperfecta types I and IV. These are rare genetic disorders and most commonly are diagnosed from a combination of the clinical findings, the family history and the radiographic features. The latter include:
    I wormian bones. These are multiple small extra bones in a mosaic distribution, seen in the sutures of the skull, usually in the lambdoid suture and posterior part of the sagittal suture. They are present in only a proportion of patients with osteogenesis imperfecta. They are usually too numerous to count. Up to 10 wormian bones may be seen as a normal variant finding
    I large anterior fontanelle
    I osteopenia
    I slender ribs
    I mild lateral bowing of the femora. This finding is only present occasionally
    I diaphyseal fractures usually occurring after the child becomes mobile and actively weight-bearing. Absence of metaphyseal fractures, periosteal shearing injuries and skull fractures.
        Rarely, there are infants with fractures where a clear diagnosis of either abuse or osteogenesis imperfecta cannot be established from the clinical/radiological findings, and screening for mutations in type IA collagen may be undertaken

to help to establish a diagnosis of osteogenesis imperfecta. It should also be remembered that both conditions might co-exist. Rare forms of osteogenesis imperfecta (usually autosomal recessive forms) may not have mutations in the type IA collagen.

- Disuse osteoporosis. In young children this usually occurs following immobilisation for an initial diaphyseal fracture. Following removal of the Plaster of Paris and active mobilisation, a further fracture may occur in the same limb. This should be recognised as disuse osteoporosis and not automatically regarded as evidence of ongoing physical abuse. Fracturing may also occur as a result of disuse osteoporosis when the Plaster of Paris is still in position, with the edge of the plaster acting as a fulcrum.
- Disuse osteoporosis also occurs in neurological conditions and in any situation where a child is wheelchair bound. Fractures occur in an older age group.
- Steroid therapy.

— Pathological fractures through localised areas of abnormal bone – either congenital or acquired.

— Abnormal stresses through normal bone occur in active children with congenital insensitivity to pain. Repeated trauma or normal activity in the presence of painless underlying fractures results in re-fracturing, bone fragmentation, exuberant callus and deformity.

5.1 FEMUR: TRANSVERSE FRACTURE

Age of fracture:	<10 days (no periosteal reaction, sharp fracture margins)
Degree of force:	Significant
Mechanism:	Direct blow May also result from indirect forces associated with swinging, levering, slamming or throwing the infant
Prevalence in abuse:	Common (up to 30%)
Specificity for abuse:	High if non-ambulant Medium/low if ambulant

➥ Femoral fractures most commonly affect the middle third of the diaphysis.
➥ Proximal fractures require a significant force and therefore in the absence of a history of trauma are more indicative of abuse.
➥ Note angulated and overlapping nature of the fracture fragments.

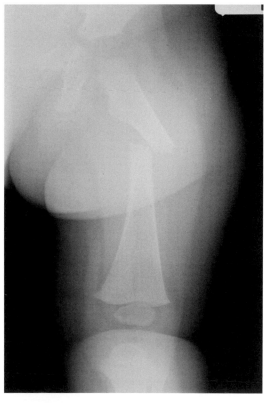

A: AP left femur

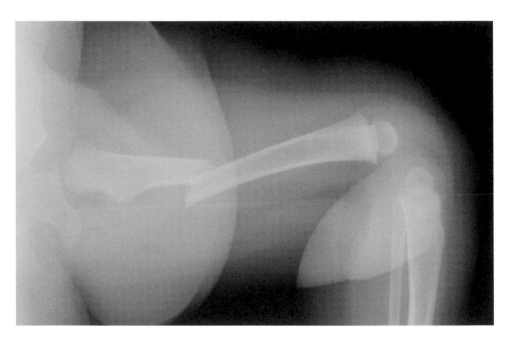

B: Lateral left femur

5.2 FEMUR: OBLIQUE/SPIRAL FRACTURE

Age of fracture:	2–4 weeks (soft callus, fracture line visible)
Degree of force:	Significant
Mechanism:	Torsional force while holding onto the affected limb Torsional force exerted at point of impact following a fall/throw
Prevalence in abuse:	Common (up to 30%)
Specificity for abuse:	High if non-ambulant Medium/low if ambulant

➥ Whether a fracture is spiral, oblique or transverse bears no relevance to whether it was inflicted or accidental – correlation with the stated mechanism is the crucial factor.

➥ A fracture may appear spiral on one view and oblique on another. These particular terms bear no relevance to the mechanism of injury.

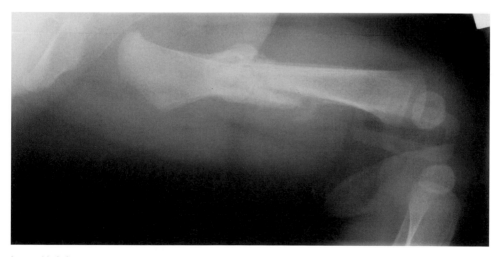

Lateral left femur

5.3 FEMUR: IMPACTED FRACTURE

Age of fracture: <10 days (no periosteal reaction, soft tissue swelling)

Degree of force: Significant

Mechanism: Direct force along the length of the bone

Prevalence in abuse: Common (up to 30%)

Specificity for abuse: High if non-ambulant
                          Medium/low if ambulant

➡ Impacted distal femoral fractures are likely to be the result of an axial force extending up the femur from a fall, with force, onto the flexed knee.

➡ Such fractures are also relatively common as pathological fractures secondary to normal handling of non-ambulant children (e.g., cerebral palsy) with osteopenic bones.

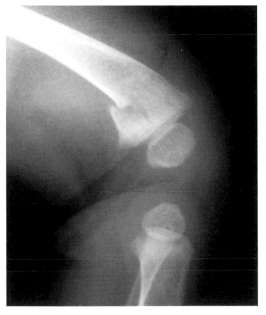

Lateral knee

5.4 TIBIA: COMPLEX FRACTURE

Age of fracture: <10 days (soft tissue swelling, sharp fracture margins)

Degree of force: Significant

Mechanism: Direct blow or levering action

Prevalence in abuse: Common (up to 30%)

Specificity for abuse: High if non-ambulant
                            Medium/low if ambulant

➡ Note that there has been a previous injury as evidenced by the periosteal reaction along the medial and lateral tibial cortices.

➡ The periosteal reaction is not related to the complex tibial fracture – the fracture line extends through the periosteal reaction (arrow). This is a case of *repetitive injury* (i.e., multiple episodes of trauma affecting a given site).

➡ The fact that two bony injuries have affected the same bone within weeks of each other could indicate that the second fracture was the result of some disuse osteoporosis. This would be more likely if the child were ambulant.

➡ *Repeated injury* indicates multiple episodes of trauma affecting different sites (as evidenced by multiple fractures of different age).

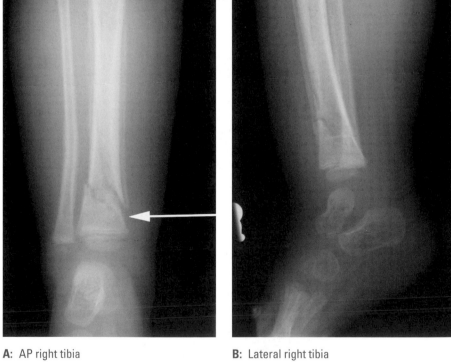

A: AP right tibia

B: Lateral right tibia

5.5 TIBIA: SUBPERIOSTEAL NEW BONE FORMATION

Age of fracture:	At least 10 days (visible calcified periosteum)
Degree of force:	Moderate
Mechanism:	Direct shearing forces stripping periosteum
Prevalence in abuse:	Unknown and probably under-reported
Specificity for abuse:	High

➥ Note that in abuse, SPNBF may occur in isolation and does not necessarily indicate an underlying fracture.
➥ SPNBF should be differentiated from physiological periosteal reaction (*see* Plates 5.14 and 9.4).
➥ The sclerotic transverse lines across the upper tibial shaft represent the anterior and posterior edges of the circumferential periosteal cuff.

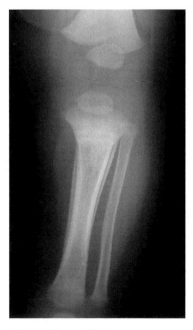

AP left tibia and fibula

5.6 FOOT, METATARSAL FRACTURES

Age of fracture:	<10 days (no healing reaction)
Degree of force:	Significant
Mechanism:	Indirect forces as the foot is forcefully gripped and squeezed Direct impact
Prevalence in abuse:	Uncommon
Specificity for abuse:	High

➥ Metatarsal fractures usually occur at the metatarsal bases.

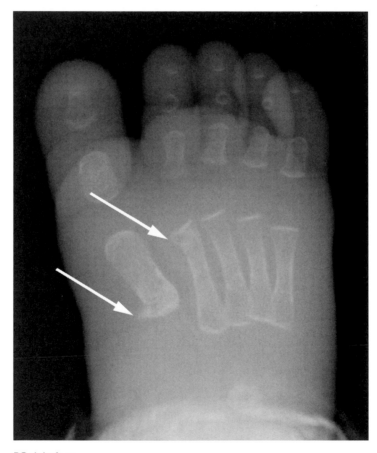

DP right foot

5.7: FOOT, METATARSAL FRACTURES

Age of fracture:	4–6 weeks (sclerosis at fracture site indicative of a healing response and indistinct fracture lines)
Degree of force:	Significant
Mechanism:	Indirect forces as the foot is gripped and squeezed Direct impact
Prevalence in abuse:	Uncommon
Specificity for abuse:	High

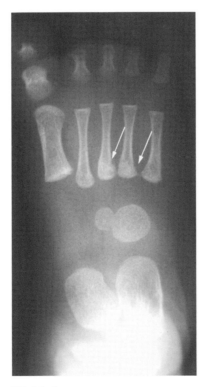

DP right foot

5.8 HUMERUS: OBLIQUE/SPIRAL FRACTURE

Age of fracture:	7–14 days (fracture line clearly visible, early periosteal reaction)
Degree of force:	Significant
Mechanism:	Torsional force while holding onto the affected limb Torsional force exerted at point of impact following a fall/throw
Prevalence in abuse:	Common (up to 40%)
Specificity for abuse:	High

➡ Most humeral fractures in abuse affect the middle/distal thirds of the shaft.

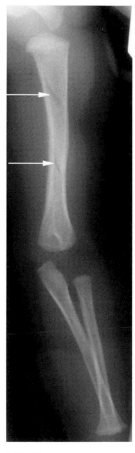

AP left humerus

5.9 HUMERUS: TRANSVERSE FRACTURE

Age of fracture:	7–14 days (early periosteal reaction, fracture line visible)
Degree of force:	Significant
Mechanism:	Indirect bending/levering force while grasping elbow/forearm Direct blow
Prevalence in abuse	Common (up to 40%)
Specificity for abuse:	High

➥ It is common (as in this case) for transverse humeral fractures to be angulated.

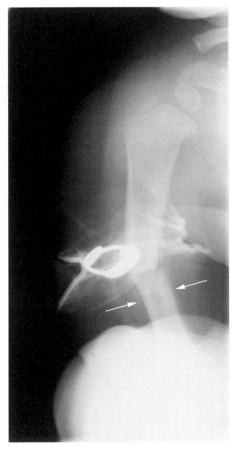

AP right humerus

5.10 HUMERUS: PROXIMAL GROWTH PLATE FRACTURE/SEPARATION

Age of fracture: <10 days (no periosteal reaction)

Degree of force: Significant

Mechanism: Complex forces involving sudden forward flexion and
                          hyperabduction of the shoulder

Prevalence in abuse: Rare

Specificity for abuse: High

➡ This is a relatively common birth-related injury.
➡ Unlike in this example, in birth trauma the humeral head and greater
  tuberosity are usually displaced laterally.

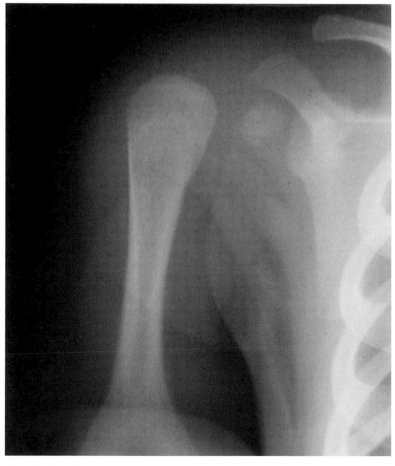

AP right shoulder

5.11 HUMERUS: LATERAL CONDYLAR FRACTURE

Age of fracture:	<10 days (significant soft tissue swelling, no periosteal reaction)
Degree of force:	Significant
Mechanism:	Hyperextension of the elbow
Prevalence in abuse:	Less common than shaft fractures
Specificity for abuse:	Medium

➥ Fractures of the distal humerus are usually supracondylar (*see* Plate 5.12) or lateral condylar as shown. True CMLs are rare at this site (*see* Plate 6.5).

➥ Note the soft tissue oedema with loss of definition of the soft tissue planes.

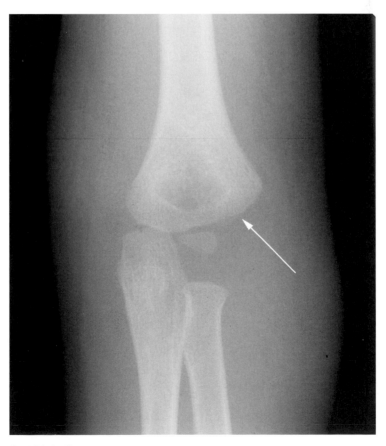

A: AP left elbow

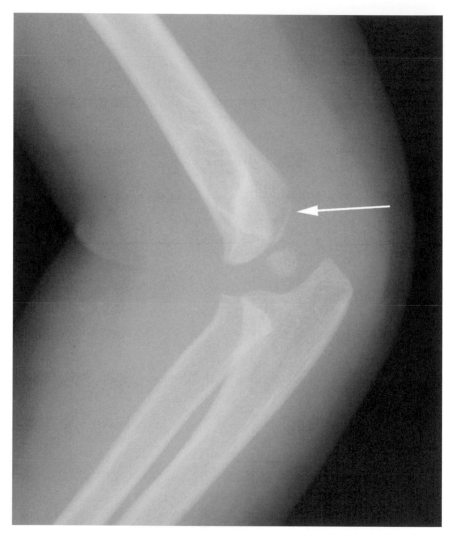

B: Lateral left elbow

5.12 HUMERUS: SUPRACONDYLAR FRACTURE

Age of fracture: <10 days (soft tissue swelling, no periosteal reaction)

Degree of force: Significant

Mechanism: Hyperextension of the elbow

Prevalence in abuse: Less common than shaft fractures

Specificity for abuse: Medium

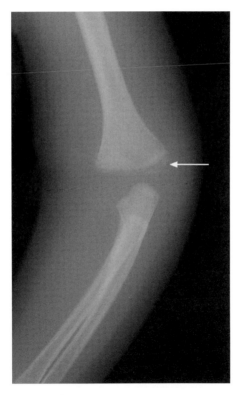

Oblique left elbow

5.13 FOREARM: TRANSVERSE FRACTURE

Age of fracture: 2–4 weeks (soft callus, fracture line visible)

Degree of force: Significant

Mechanism: Indirect angular force while holding distal forearm/hand
Direct blow as a child (in an older age group) attempts to defend him- or herself

Prevalence in abuse: Up to 20%

Specificity for abuse: Medium (high in non-ambulant child)

➥ The injury demonstrated (transverse fractures of the radius and ulna at the same level) is termed a *nightstick* injury.

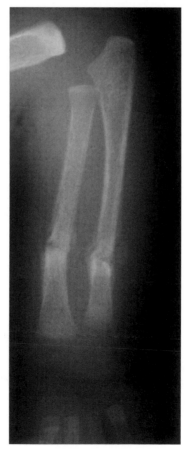

A: AP forearm

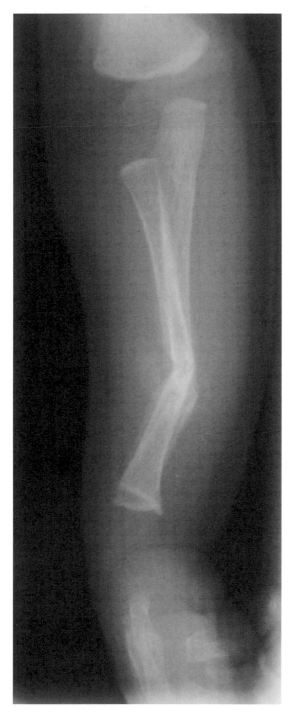

B: Lateral forearm

5.14 FOREARM: SUPERIOSTEAL NEW BONE FORMATION

Age of fracture: At least 10 days (visible calcified periosteum)

Degree of force: Moderate

Mechanism: Direct shearing forces stripping periosteum

Prevalence in abuse: Unknown and probably under-reported

Specificity for abuse: High

➡ Note that in abuse, SPNBF may occur in isolation and does not
  necessarily indicate an underlying fracture.
➡ SPNBF should be differentiated from physiological periosteal reaction
  (*see* Plates 5.5 and 9.4).

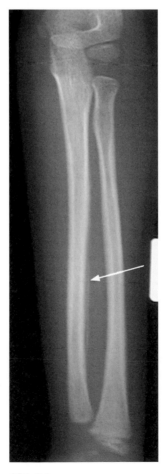

AP left forearm

5.15 HAND: METACARPAL FRACTURE

Age of fracture: 6–8 weeks (hard callus, fracture line not visible)

Degree of force: Significant

Mechanism: Twisting/bending or gripping/squeezing forces

Prevalence in abuse: Uncommon (<3%)

Specificity for abuse: High

➡ The second and third metacarpals are said to be those most commonly injured in abuse.

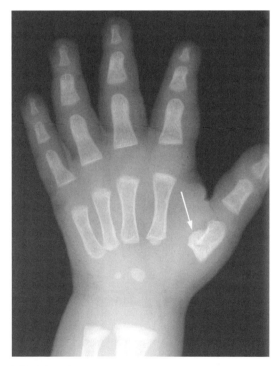

DP left hand

CHAPTER 6

Classical metaphyseal lesions (CMLs)

CMLs are seen in infants at the ends of the long bones, immediately adjacent to the growth plate (physis). Histologically, a thin transverse plate of bone is detached from the adjacent metaphysis. Radiologically, this is seen as a circumferential rim because of the relatively thicker metaphyseal 'cuff', rather than as a plate of bone. Depending on the position of the limb in relation to the X-ray beam, the metaphyseal fracture may be given various descriptive terms relating to the radiographic appearance. It may be referred to as 'bucket-handle' when a rim of part of the circumference of the metaphyseal fracture is seen lifted from the adjacent metaphysis. Alternatively it may be described as 'corner-fracture' when the rim is seen more tangentially. These descriptions both refer to CMLs and the same fracture may appear as 'bucket-handle' or 'corner fracture' depending on the radiographic projection and the angle of the X-ray beam. The most common sites of involvement are the knees, wrists and ankles, but any metaphysis may be injured.

MECHANISMS OF CAUSATION

CMLs are thought to result from the direct application, simultaneously, of gripping, twisting and pulling forces (torsion and traction) at the sites of the fractures. It has also been suggested that CMLs may occur during the course of a shaking episode. In this situation the limbs flail about and during this process may generate the appropriately severe tractional and torsional forces. This is likely to be an uncommon mechanism of causation of metaphyseal fractures. Typically they are not usually associated with overlying soft tissue changes in the form of swelling or oedema and may not be apparent on clinical examination of the infant. They are sometimes referred to as being clinically silent.

CML HEALING

CMLs may or may not be associated with periosteal new bone formation as part of the healing process. Commonly the periosteum is not damaged during the application of force, because it does not extend to the very ends of the bone. In this situation a periosteal reaction and callus do not form and the fracture heals by a process of gradual consolidation to the adjacent bone. Typically the healing process is radiologically complete in four weeks. The fracture line becomes indistinct from the end of the first week and cannot be identified by about four weeks. With relatively greater forces, or when forces are applied over a larger area, damage to the periosteum will occur in addition to the CML. This will result in some periosteal new bone formation seen extending along the metadiaphyseal shaft after one week. Subsequently a small amount of callus may be present. This type of CML will take longer than four weeks to resolve radiologically.

EFFECT OF CMLs

— Pain, as soon as the fractures occur, resulting in the demonstration of pain, e.g., excessive crying.
— Ongoing pain for several days following the fractures on any direct handling of the injured area, resulting in further demonstration of pain. This may not be localised by the regular carers and may be put down to other childhood ailments.
— Typically no swelling or bruising.
— Normal movements of the injured limb.

Differential diagnosis is required from some medical conditions and from normal variants. They may show varying degrees of metaphyseal irregularity and marginal spurs. These will all show symmetrical changes and affect many areas of the skeleton. Typically the most florid changes will be seen in areas which are growing most rapidly – adjacent to the knees and the wrists. The bucket-handle appearance is seen only with CMLs.

— Osteopathy (bone disease) of prematurity is found in some infants delivered before 33 weeks gestation of less than 1.5 kg in weight and who have had complications relating to prematurity, sometimes requiring parenteral nutrition. The bone changes include a metabolic bone disease with osteopenia, frayed metaphyses and periosteal reactions. There is a generalised coarsening of the trabecular pattern. The changes are not present after the age of 6 months.
— Rickets shows flared and irregular metaphyses. It is unusual in infancy unless seen as part of severe renal disease.
— Scurvy is extremely rare in Western cultures but results in osteopenia (the pencil outline of the epiphyses or Wimberger's sign) and spurs at the metaphyses. These are known as Pelcan spurs and typically point at right angles to the axis of the long bone unlike the CMLs associated with abuse.
— Metaphyseal (spondylo) chondrodysplasias have flared, irregular metaphyses, but they are not usually apparent in infancy and are symmetrical.
— Normal variants include small marginal spurs at the metaphyses in the rapidly growing infant. These may cause confusion with small corner-fractures. Additional views may be necessary to demonstrate the true rim (bucket-handle) appearance of a fracture or to demonstrate that the normal spurs are still present four weeks after the initial radiographs when CMLs would have healed.
— True CMLs may occur in acute osteomyelitis and septic arthritis. The precise relationship of the two is unclear. CMLs (as a result of physical abuse) may form the focus for infection in an already septic infant. Alternatively, multifocal osteomyelitis may result in sufficient localised bone weakening for normal handling to result in CMLs. The coexistence of multifocal osteomyelitis and CMLs is extremely rare and raises the possibility of abuse in the presence of sepsis.

6.1 CML: PROXIMAL FEMUR

Age of fracture:	<4 weeks (irregularity remains visible)
Degree of force:	High
Mechanism:	Gripping, twisting and pulling – perhaps during the course of nappy changing
Prevalence in abuse:	Rare
Specificity for abuse:	High

➥ In the correct clinical setting, CMLs are pathognomonic of abuse.

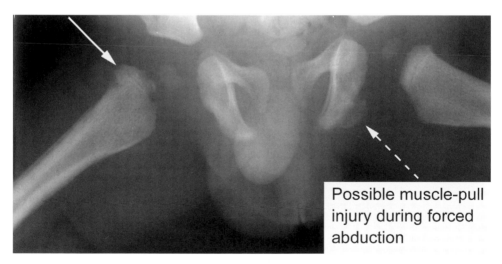

Possible muscle-pull injury during forced abduction

AP pelvis

6.2 CML: DISTAL FEMUR

Age of fracture: <4 weeks (fracture clearly visible)

Degree of force: Moderate

Mechanism: Torsional/tractional forces as limb is twisted
                     and pulled

Prevalence in abuse: Up to 24%

Specificity for abuse: High

➡ A periosteal reaction is not usually seen with healing of metaphyseal
  fractures.
➡ The periosteal reaction seen on this radiograph is indicative of damage/
  shearing injury to the periosteum at the time of the trauma.
➡ The upper tibia has several growth arrest lines (Park's lines). These may
  be seen in infants who are the subject of physical abuse with associated
  neglect.

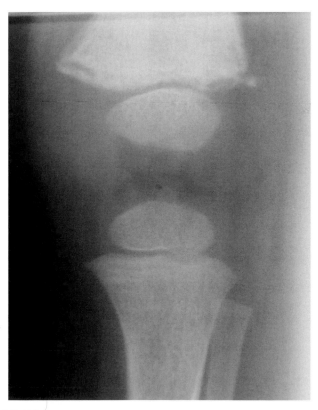

A: AP knee

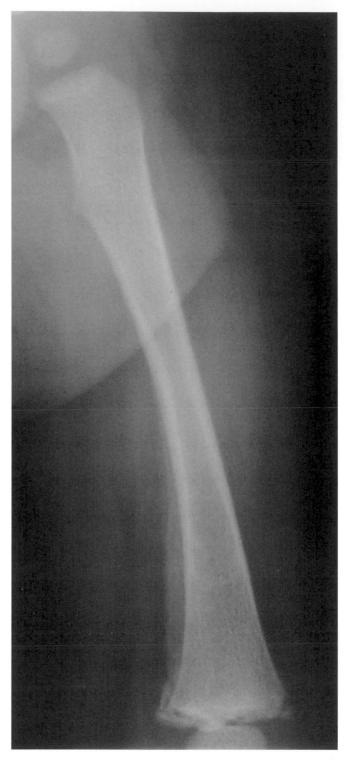

B: AP femur

6.3 CML: PROXIMAL TIBIA

Age of fracture: <4 weeks (fracture line remains visible)

Degree of force: High

Mechanism: Torsional/tractional forces as limb is twisted and pulled

Prevalence in abuse: Common

Specificity for abuse: High

➡ Note also the CMLs of the distal femur and distal tibia.
➡ Note that the same fracture may have a bucket-handle or corner-fracture appearance, depending on projection. These terms are descriptive only and are of no significance as regards mechanism of injury, fracture dating, etc.

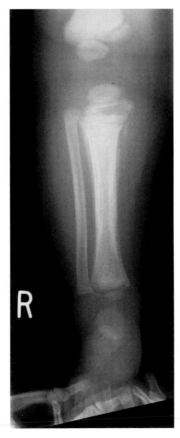

A: AP right knee

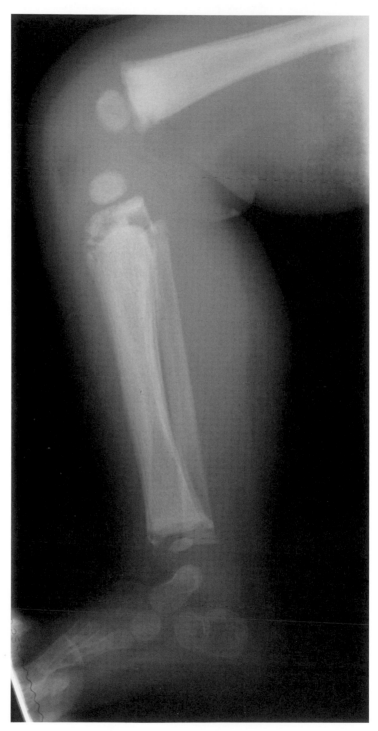

B: Lateral right knee

6.4 CML: DISTAL TIBIA

Age of fracture: <4 weeks (fracture lines still visible)

Degree of force: Moderate

Mechanism: Torsional/tractional forces as limb is twisted and pulled

Prevalence in abuse: Common

Specificity for abuse: High

➡ The distal femur, proximal tibia and distal tibia are the commonest sites of CMLs in abuse.
➡ Notice also the CMLs of the right proximal fibula and left proximal tibia (arrows).

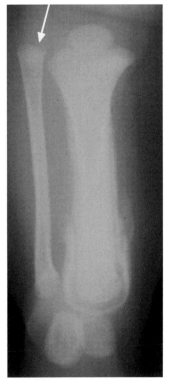

A: AP right tibia and fibula

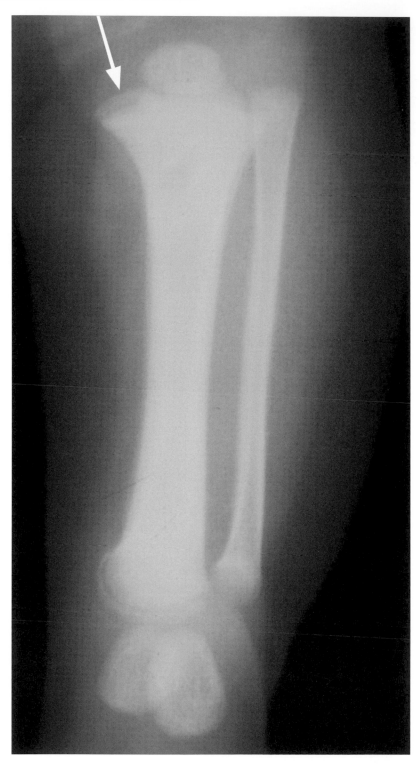

B: AP left tibia and fibula

6.5 CML: PROXIMAL HUMERUS

Age of fracture:	<4 weeks
Degree of force:	High
Mechanism:	Torsional/tractional forces as limb is twisted and pulled
Prevalence in abuse:	Uncommon
Specificity for abuse:	High

- ➡ There is also a supracondylar fracture of the distal humerus.
- ➡ True metaphyseal fractures of the distal humerus are rare at this age (*see* Plate 5.11).
- ➡ Note irregular periosteal reaction of the proximal ulna, suggesting an associated injury of this bone.
- ➡ Images B (at presentation) and C (three weeks later) show progressive periosteal reaction in another child with a proximal humeral CML.

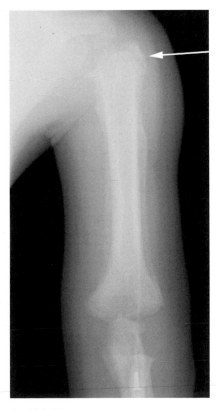

A: AP left humerus

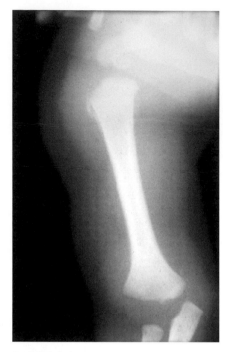

B: AP right humerus

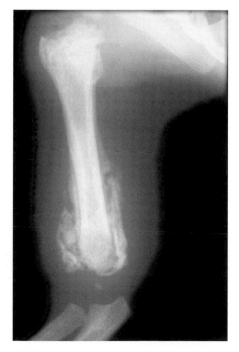

C: AP right humerus

6.6 CML: DISTAL RADIUS/ULNA

Age of fracture:	<4 weeks (fracture lines remain visible)
Degree of force:	Moderate
Mechanism:	Torsional/tractional forces as limb is twisted and pulled
Prevalence in abuse:	Fairly common
Specificity for abuse:	High

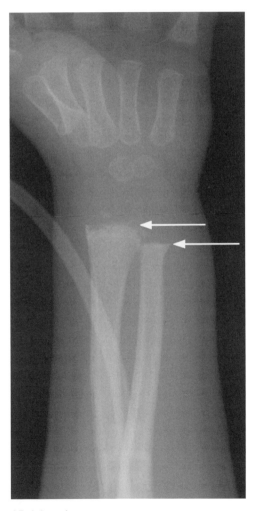

AP right wrist

CHAPTER 7

Visceral injuries

Intra-abdominal injury results from blunt trauma to the abdomen. It is more commonly seen in an older, toddler age group. The association with anterior costochondral junction rib fractures has already been described and is the result of a direct blow to the epigastrium. The trauma may result in laceration of a solid organ, most commonly the liver, pancreas or spleen with intra-abdominal bleeding. Alternatively a hollow viscus may perforate. This may be the bladder or any part of the bowel. Typically the duodenum perforates due to its more vulnerable fixed retroperitoneal position overlying the spine. Bowel perforation commonly results in peritonitis and is associated with a high mortality.

Other intra-abdominal injuries include mesenteric tears and haematomas of the bowel wall, which may cause obstruction.

Bleeding from any orifice is extremely unusual in infancy. In the absence of a bleeding disorder it is often suggestive of some form of physical or sexual abuse.

- Bleeding from the mouth may result from an inappropriate object being forced into the mouth causing oral or pharyngeal lacerations. This may result in a mediastinitis, mediastinal or surgical emphysema, or pneumothorax and respiratory distress.
- Bleeding from the rectum is usually the result of anal tears and may be put down to constipation, but sexual abuse is a recognised cause.
- Bleeding from the nose in infants, in the absence of a severe upper respiratory tract infection, may be a sign of attempted suffocation.

7.1 VISCERAL INJURY: MULTIPLE SUBCUTANEOUS FOREIGN BODIES

Age of injury: Dating is not possible

Degree of force: Not relevant

Mechanism: Foreign body insertion

Prevalence in abuse: Rare

Specificity for abuse: High

➥ This 3-year-old girl's infant sibling (also female) died from a cerebral abscess. Post-mortem examination revealed an intracerebral needle.
➥ Notice on the CT (B) how one needle just misses the great vessels of the neck.
➥ Notice further needles overlying other regions (C–E).
➥ This family from the Indian sub-continent did not want girls.
➥ Do not confuse abuse with other cultural practices that may involve acupuncture.

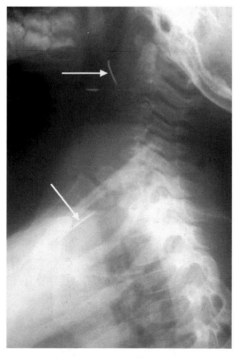

A: Lateral cervical spine

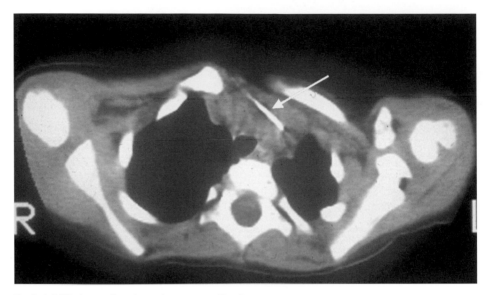

B: Axial CT chest: slice through upper mediastinum

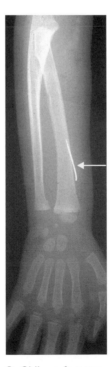

C: Oblique, forearm

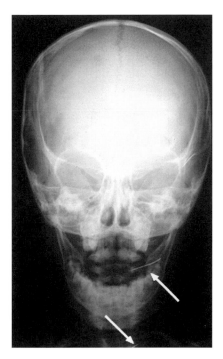

D: AP skull

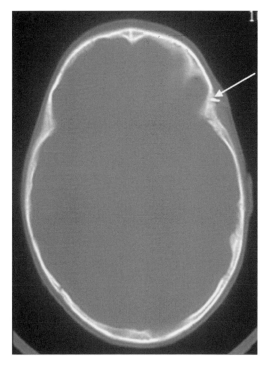

E: Axial CT head, bone window

7.2 VISCERAL INJURY: MULTIPLE SUBCUTANEOUS FOREIGN BODIES

Age of injury: Dating is not possible

Degree of force: Not relevant

Mechanism: Foreign body insertion

Prevalence in abuse: Rare

Specificity for abuse: High

➥ Premature neonate on NICU.
➥ Two needles were initially thought to be artefacts outside the neonate (A).
➥ Two weeks later, four needles were present (B). Mother had rejected her baby and admitted inserting the needles.

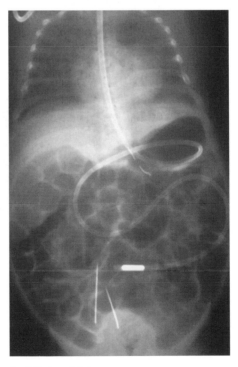

A: AP chest/abdomen

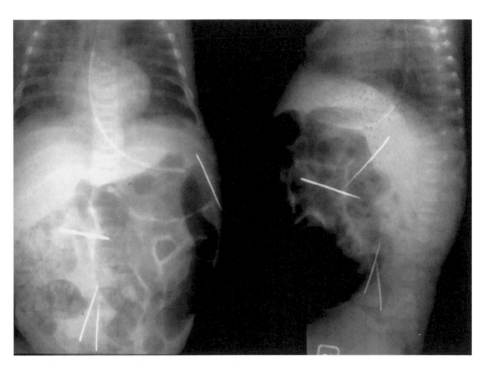

B: AP & lateral chest/abdomen

7.3 VISCERAL INJURY: PHARYNGEAL PERFORATION WITH RETROPHARYNGEAL ABSCESS

Age of injury:	Not possible to date
Degree of force:	Not relevant
Mechanism:	Foreign body insertion
Prevalence in abuse:	Rare
Specificity for abuse:	High

➥ Note anterior deviation of airways by soft tissue mass.
➥ Oral contrast (arrow) does not follow the path of the nasogastric tube, indicating perforation.
➥ This infant later presented with multiple skeletal injuries.

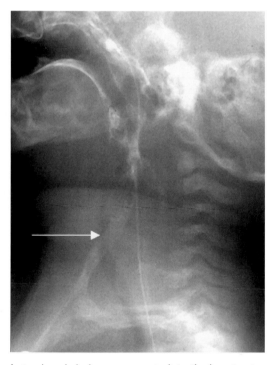

Lateral neck during upper gastrointestinal contrast study

7.4 VISCERAL INJURY: RUPTURED HOLLOW VISCUS AND ANTERIOR RIB FRACTURES

Age of injury:	Acute. This infant was brought in dead, and had a skeletal survey as part of the work-up for sudden unexpected death in infancy
Degree of force:	Significant
Mechanism:	Blunt abdominal trauma
Prevalence in abuse:	Rare (<10%, but may be under-reported)
Specificity for abuse:	High (in infants)

➡ Rupture of a hollow viscus is the commonest injury associated with abdominal trauma in abuse.
➡ Inflicted visceral injuries are more common in toddlers and older children.
➡ Free intraperitoneal air in association with fractures of the lower ribs is a relatively common combination.
➡ Post-mortem examination revealed a duodenal tear.
➡ *See* Plates 7.5 and 8.10.

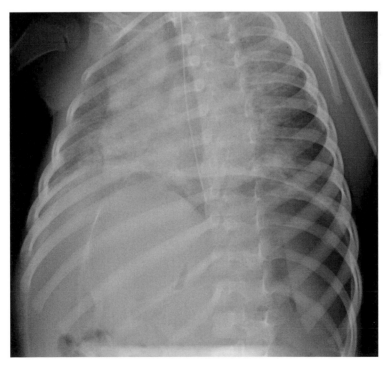

Chest radiographs
A: Right oblique

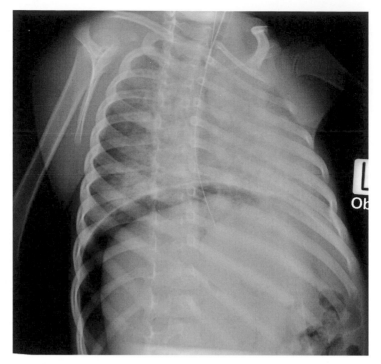

B: Left oblique

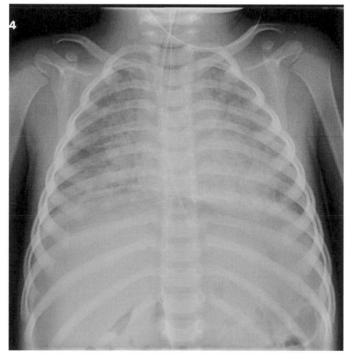

C: AP

7.5 VISCERAL INJURY: RUPTURED HOLLOW VISCUS AND ANTERIOR RIB FRACTURES

Age of injury:	Acute. This infant was brought in dead, and had a skeletal survey as part of the work-up for sudden unexpected death in infancy
Degree of force:	Significant
Mechanism:	Blunt abdominal trauma
Prevalence in abuse:	Rare (<10%, but may be under-reported)
Specificity for abuse:	High (in infants)

➡ Post-mortem examination revealed a perforated duodenum.
➡ NB Note that a babygram was performed (the image has been cropped for publishing purposes). Although the anterior rib fracture is visible (arrow), this sort of imaging is to be discouraged.
➡ *See* Plates 7.4 and 8.10.

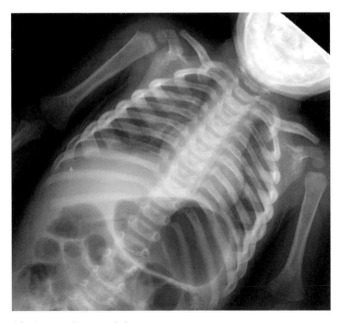

AP chest and upper abdomen

7.6 VISCERAL INJURY: PANCREATIC PSEUDOCYST

Age of injury:	Dating not possible
Degree of force:	Significant
Mechanism:	Blunt abdominal trauma
Prevalence in abuse:	Rare (<10%, but may be under-reported)
Specificity for abuse:	High (in infants and toddlers)

➥ Note the pancreatic laceration (solid arrow) with resultant pancreatic pseudocyst (dashed arrow).
➥ This child also had acute costochondral fractures of the lower ribs (*see* Plate 3.8).

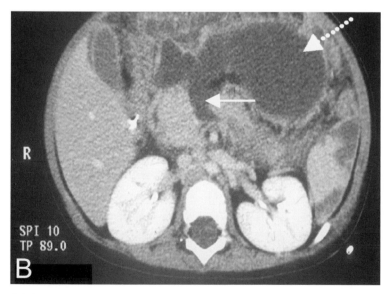

Axial contrast enhanced CT scan – slice at level of renal hilae

7.7 VISCERAL INJURY: SUBACUTE BOWEL OBSTRUCTION

Age of injury: Dating not possible

Degree of force: Not relevant

Mechanism: Blunt abdominal trauma

Prevalence in abuse: Uncommon

Specificity for abuse: High

➡ At surgery there was a tear in the mesentery and haematoma in the adjacent bowel wall resulting in partial ileal obstruction.
➡ Notice the dilated small bowel loops and healing right femoral and right rib fractures on the abdominal radiograph.
➡ Notice the dilated ileal loops on the small bowel enema indicating the level of the partial obstruction.
➡ This 6-month-old infant had originally been diagnosed with osteogenesis imperfecta.
➡ Two months following surgery the infant was brought in dead.

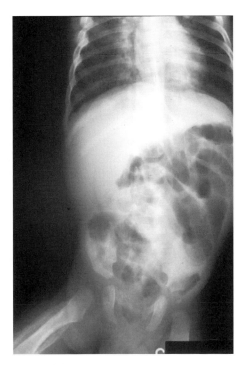

A: AP abdomen

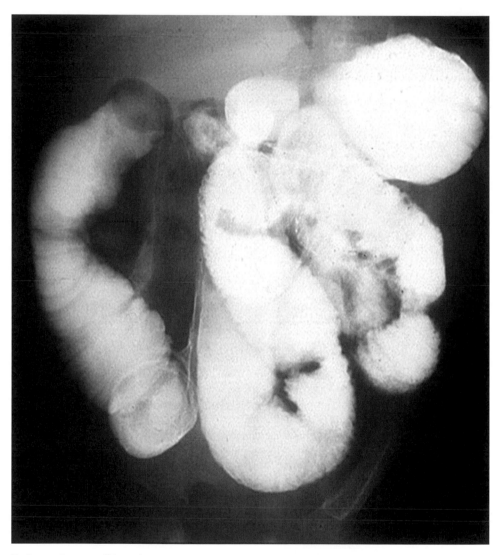

B: Image from small bowel enema

7.8 VISCERAL INJURY: DUODENAL PERFORATION

Age of injury:	Acute perforation
Degree of force:	Significant
Mechanism:	Caused by the mother's boyfriend standing on the abdomen 'as a game'
Prevalence in abuse:	Rare
Specificity for abuse:	High

- ➡ Six-year-old child.
- ➡ Lethal acute perforation from a duodenal rupture presenting 48 hours after trauma.
- ➡ Notice the old spiral fracture of the femur caused by being swung out of a 1st floor window by the mother's boyfriend.

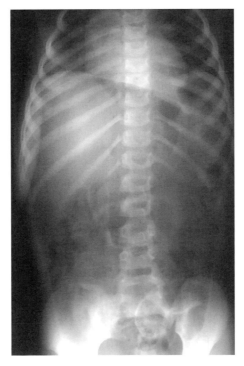

A: AP abdomen

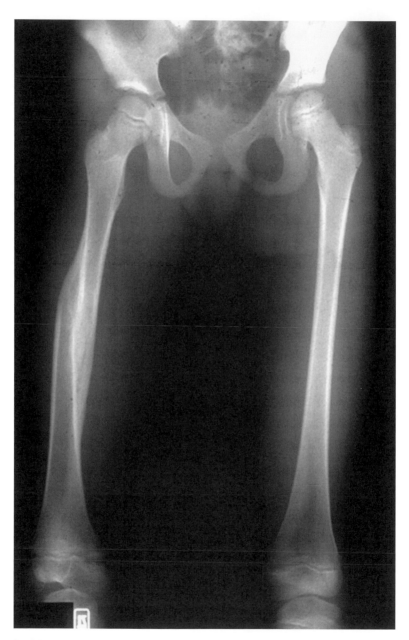

B: AP femora

7.9 VISCERAL INJURY: RECTAL PERFORATION

Age of injury:	Acute
Degree of force:	Significant
Mechanism:	Sexual abuse by mother's boyfriend
Prevalence in abuse:	Rare (<10%, but may be under-reported)
Specificity for abuse:	High (in infants and young children)

➡ This 5-year-old child presented with an acute abdomen.
➡ Figure A demonstrates signs of free intraperitoneal air:
  ▶ positive Rigler's sign – dotted arrow (air both sides of bowel wall)
  ▶ outline of falciform ligament – arrow heads (air both sides of ligament).
➡ Notice the healing fractures of both suprapubic rami (arrows) raising the distinct possibility of ongoing sexual abuse in this child.
➡ Notice the dilated loops of bowel indicating ileus.
➡ This child also had an untreated healing fracture of the humerus (Figure B).
➡ *See* Plates 4.8 and 8.3.

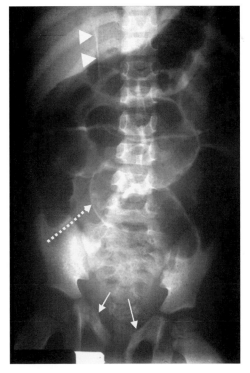

A: AP abdomen

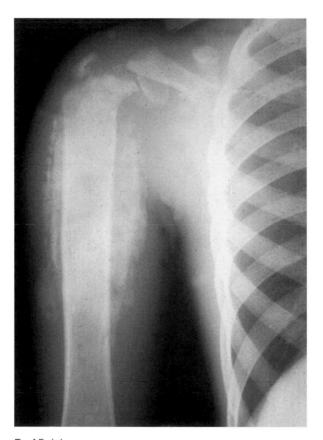

B: AP right arm

CHAPTER 8

Normal variants

8.1 PARIETAL FISSURE

➥ Also called the parietal incisura.
➥ A thin cleft in one or both parietal bones that may extend laterally from the sagittal suture for up to 10 mm or more.
➥ This remnant of the embryonic parietal notch usually disappears shortly after birth.
➥ Prevalence in the region of 1%.[91]

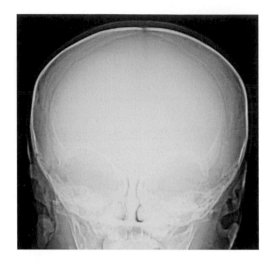

A: AP skull

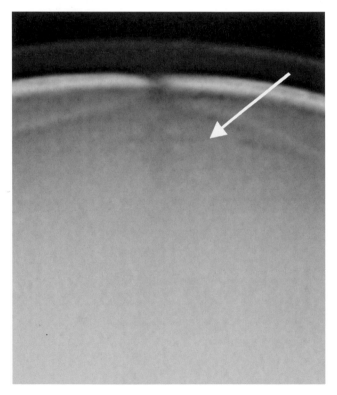

B: AP skull, coned & magnified

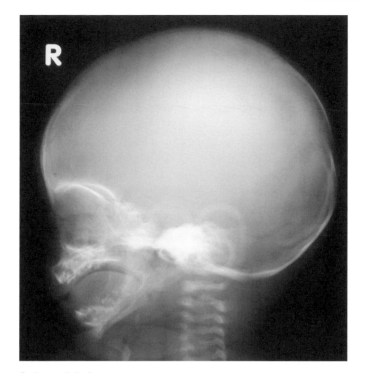

C: Lateral skull

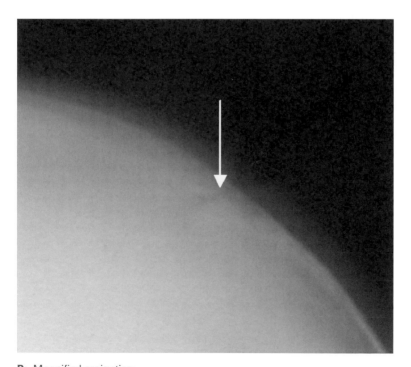

D: Magnified projection

8.2 STERNAL SEGMENTS

➥ Left and right oblique chest radiographs should be part of the routine skeletal survey (no published data to support this).

➥ *Research question: What is the effectiveness/cost effectiveness of routine oblique chest radiographs for the detection of rib fractures in suspected abuse?*

➥ Sternal segments overlying the ribs should not be mistaken for healing fractures (arrows).

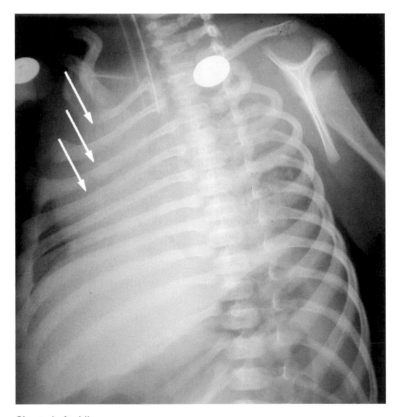

Chest: Left oblique

8.3 SUPERIOR PUBIC SYNCHONDROSIS

➡ The sclerotic line along the left superior pubic ramus represents a normal synchondrosis.

➡ This abused infant has an acute posterior fracture of the 8th rib (dashed arrow).

➡ *See* Plate 4.8.

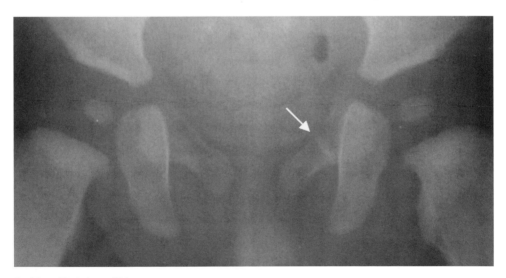

A: Magnified view of hips

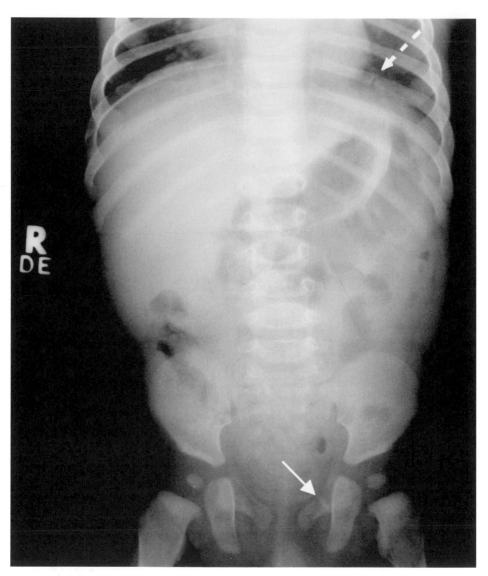

B: AP abdomen

8.4 TIBIAL CORTICAL IRREGULARITY

➡ These are bilaterally symmetrical and represent the sites of muscle attachments.
➡ It is in this position that traction spurs (small exostoses) develop in some older children.
➡ Do not confuse cortical irregularities/spurs for buckle fractures.

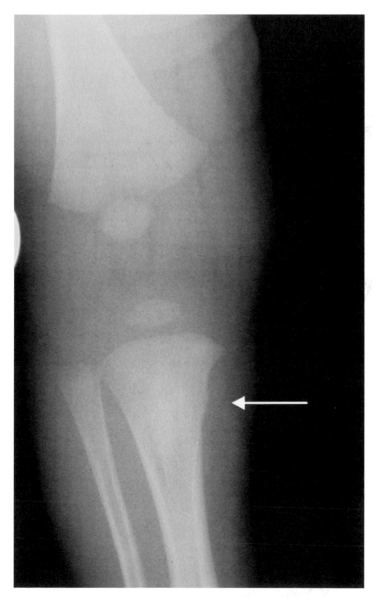

AP right knee

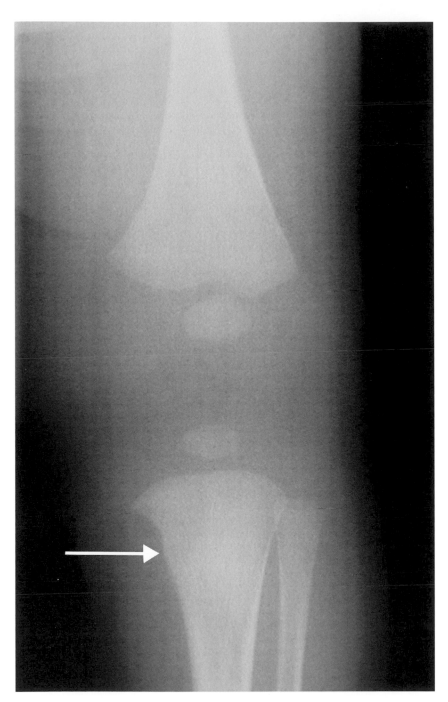

AP left knee

8.5 INTRAOSSEOUS NEEDLE TRACT

- ➡ Intraosseous needles are used to administer drugs/fluid during resuscitation.
- ➡ The tract left once they have been removed (solid arrow) should not be mistaken for a fracture.
- ➡ If in doubt review the clinical records/speak to the clinical team.
- ➡ Note the metaphyseal spurs (*see* Plate 8.7) and physiological periosteal reaction (*see* Plate 9.4).

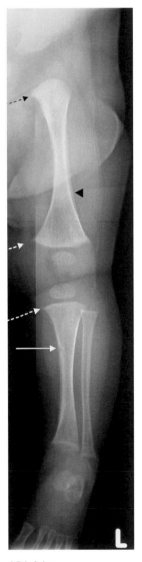

AP left leg

8.6 METACARPAL STEP

➡ Metacarpal steps affect the metacarpal heads (fractures more commonly affect the bases).

➡ Steps are bilateral and symmetrical – in this case involving metacarpals 2–4 bilaterally.

➡ They result from the obliquity of the metacarpal heads to the X-ray beam, showing anterior and posterior borders at different levels.

➡ If in doubt, there will be no significant change when comparing two radiographs obtained two weeks apart.

➡ Note also metaphyseal spur and ulna cupping (*see* Plates 8.7 and 8.9 respectively).

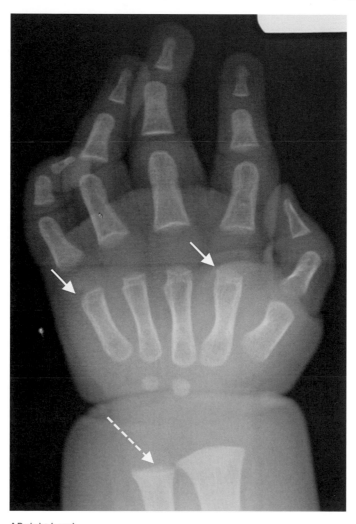

AP right hand

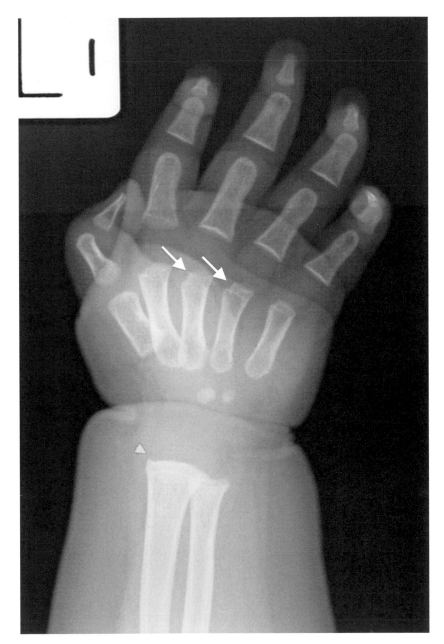

AP left hand

8.7 METAPHYSEAL SPUR

➡ Metaphyseal spurs are bilaterally symmetrical and will not change significantly when comparing two radiographs obtained two weeks apart.
➡ A fracture line will not be visible on any projection.
➡ They are seen in rapidly growing areas of the infant skeleton.

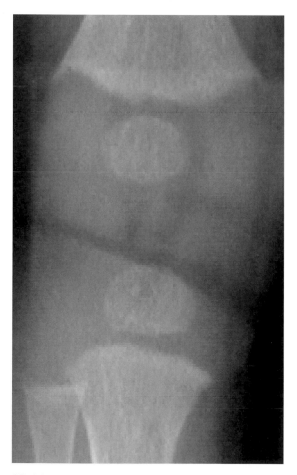

AP right knee

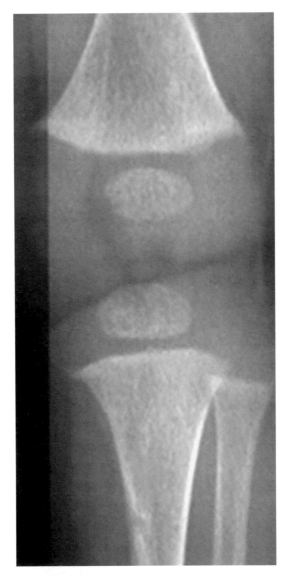

AP left knee

8.8 METAPHYSEAL LINES

➡ Metaphyseal lines are bilaterally symmetrical and will not change significantly when comparing two radiographs obtained two weeks apart.
➡ They do not extend across the width of the bone (from cortex to cortex).
➡ A fracture line will not be visible on any projection.
➡ They are growth arrest lines and may be seen following recurrent illnesses or in chronically neglected infants.

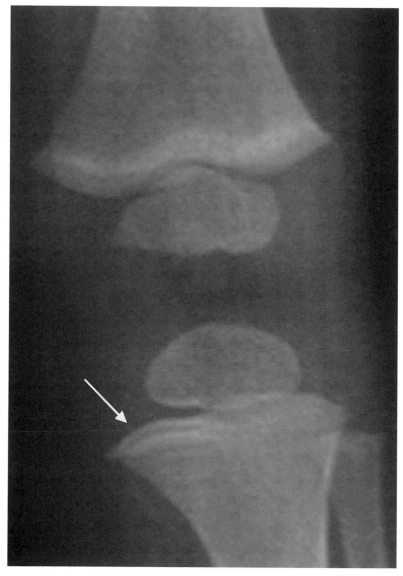

AP left knee

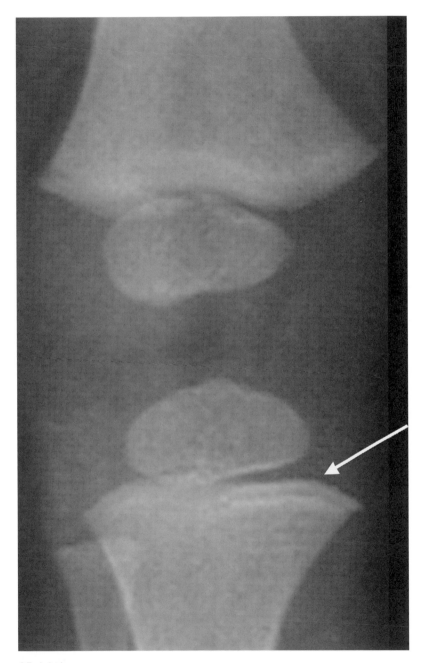

AP right knee

8.9 METAPHYSEAL CUPPING

➥ Note cupping of distal ulnar metaphysis.
➥ Metaphyseal cupping is bilaterally symmetrical and will not change significantly when comparing two radiographs obtained two weeks apart.

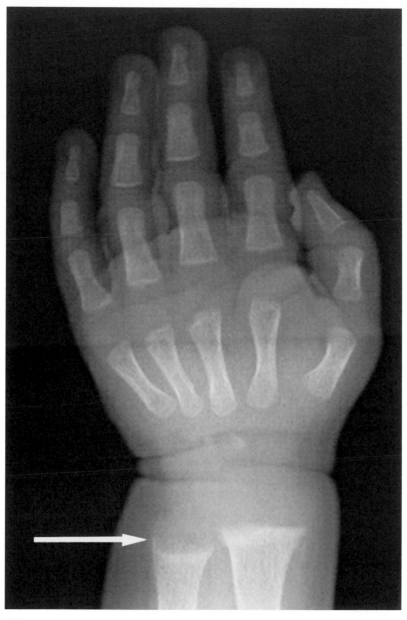

DP left hand

8.10 POST-MORTEM CHANGE

➡ Note air in the biliary tree and apparent free air around the stomach.

➡ This, in association with the anterior rib fractures (arrows) led to the diagnosis of visceral injury; however this was not confirmed at post-mortem examination.

   ◗ Both free intraperitoneal air and biliary air may occur as normal post-mortem phenomena.

➡ *See* Plates 7.4 and 7.5.

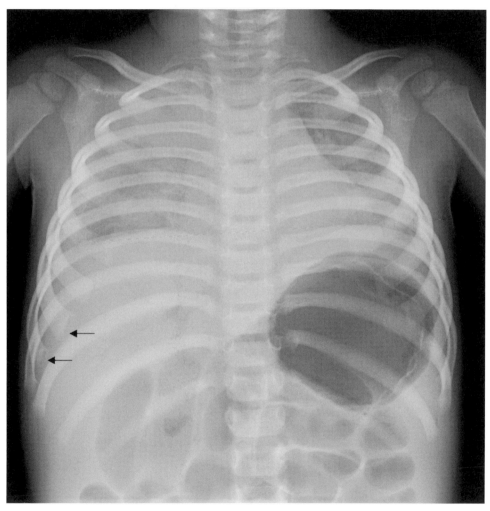

AP chest

CHAPTER 9

Pathological conditions

9.1 CEPHALHAEMATOMA CYST

➡ This results from extrinsic compression by an old cephalhaematoma.
➡ It should not be confused with a growing fracture, a depressed fracture or a 'ping-pong' fracture.
➡ *See* Plate 9.3.

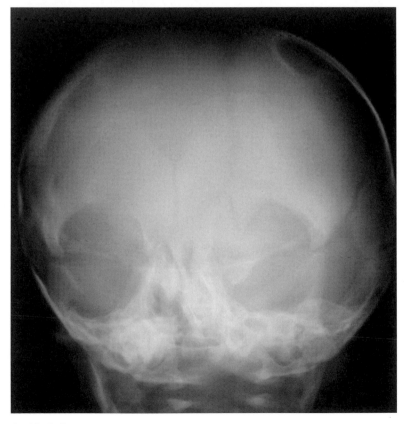

A: AP skull

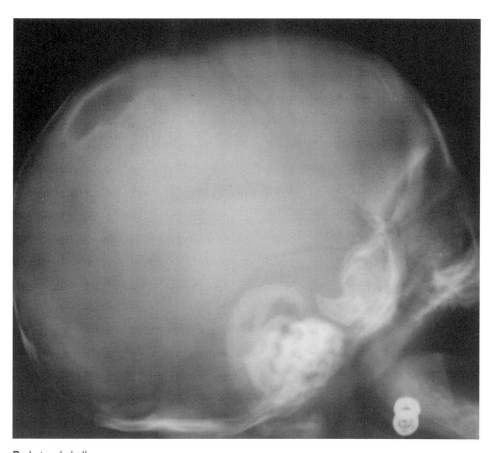

B: Lateral skull

9.2 FALSE NEGATIVE: 'WORMIAN BONES'

➥ Misdiagnosed as several wormian bones with correctly identified right parietal fractures.

➥ However, because of the earlier normal skull radiograph (not initially available to the reporting radiologist) these were in fact multiple fissured occipital fractures.

➥ Note that wormian bones are present from birth and do not subsequently appear (or disappear).

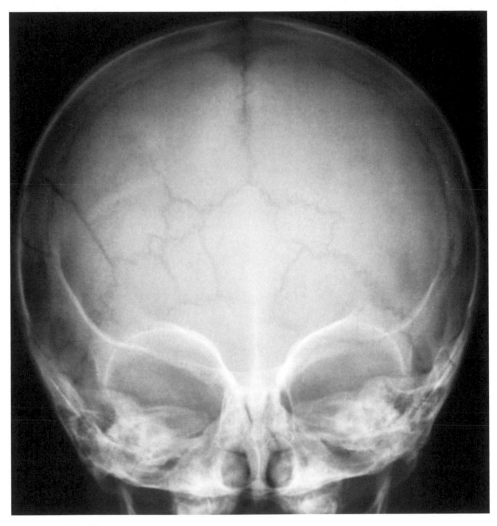

A: AP skull (April)

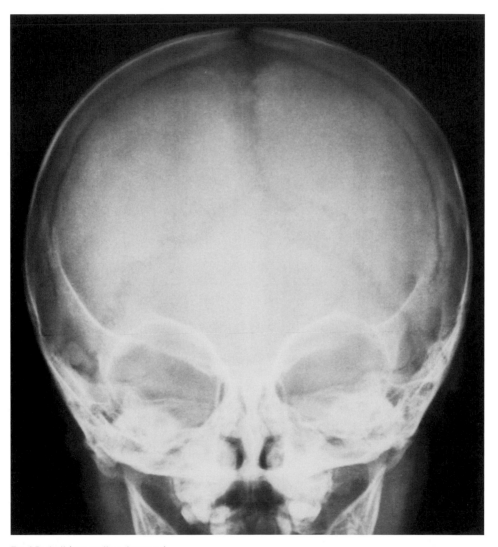

B: AP skull (preceding January)

9.3 FALSE NEGATIVE: 'INTRAUTERINE COMPRESSION'

➥ This 'ping pong' fracture was misdiagnosed as intrauterine compression due to oligohydramnios and faulty fetal packing.

➥ To differentiate the two, note the small fracture line in the centre of the depressed area on the lateral projection (arrow).

➥ *See* Plate 9.1.

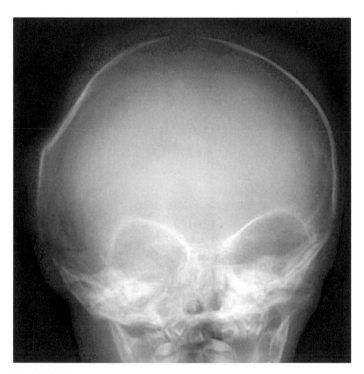

A: AP skull

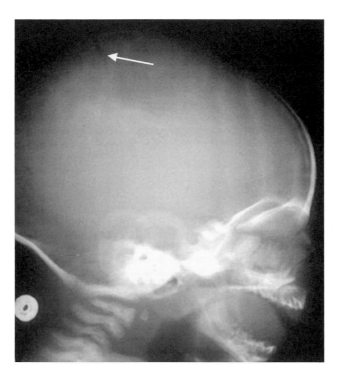

B: Lateral skull

9.4 PERIOSTEAL REACTION

➥ Physiological periosteal reaction (shown in corresponding image) is:
  ▶ seen between 4 weeks and 4 months of age
  ▶ ≤2 mm thick
  ▶ usually symmetrical and
  ▶ does not extend to the metaphyses.
➥ Causes of pathological periosteal reaction include:
  ▶ trauma (abuse or accidental)
  ▶ infection (osteomyelitis, congenital syphilis)
  ▶ metabolic (rickets, scurvy)
  ▶ tumour (leukaemia, neuroblastoma)
  ▶ iatrogenic (prostaglandin E)
  ▶ idiopathic/genetic (Caffey's disease)
  ▶ Vitamin A toxicity.
➥ Note the distal metaphyseal spurs (arrows).
➥ *See* Plate 8.7.
➥ *See also* Plates 5.5 and 5.14.

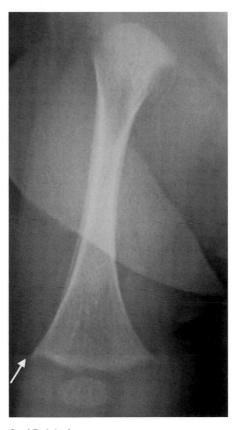

A: AP right femur

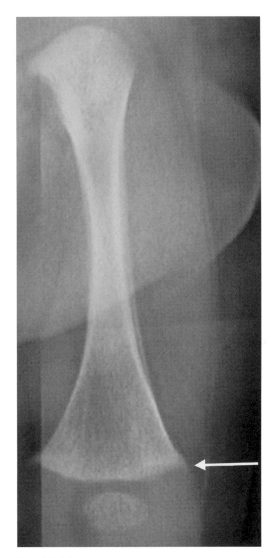

B: AP left femur

9.5 OSTEOGENESIS IMPERFECTA

➥ Generalised reduction in bone density.
➥ Multiple wormian bones (A).
  ▶ Finding ≤10 wormian bones in any given individual is within normal limits.
➥ Wide open anterior fontanelle (A).
➥ Slender 'ribbon' (B, C) or 'beaded' ribs.
➥ Broad ribs if multiple contiguous fractures have occurred.
➥ Bowed long bones (C, D).
➥ Multiple fractures (ribs, long bones, vertebrae).
  ▶ Skull and metaphyseal fractures are uncommon presentations of OI.
➥ Family history/clinical features.
➥ Types of OI:
  ▶ I: of relatively mild severity (A = DI*, B = no DI), blue sclerae
  ▶ II: perinatally lethal (sharp angulation of tibiae)
  ▶ III: most severe non-lethal type (unlikely to be misdiagnosed as abuse), blue sclerae
  ▶ IV: of relatively moderate severity (A = DI, B = no DI), white sclerae
  ▶ other types are rare.
➥ In types I and IV, frequency of fractures decreases with age.
➥ Remember that a child with OI may also have been abused.

* DI = dentinogenesis imperfecta

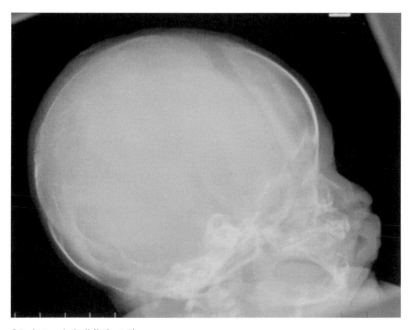

A1: Lateral skull (Infant 1)

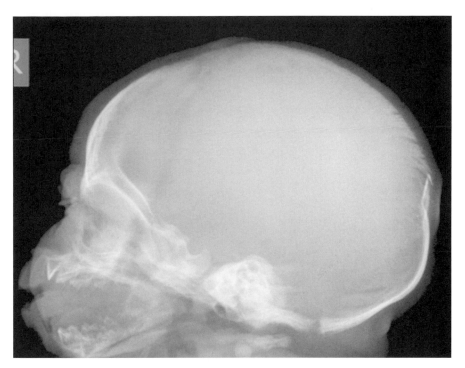

A2: Lateral skull (Infant 2)

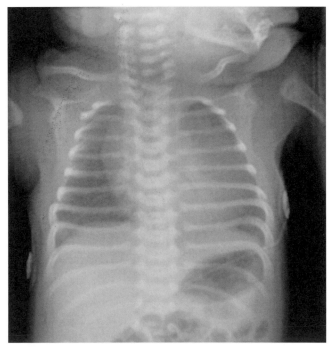

B: AP chest

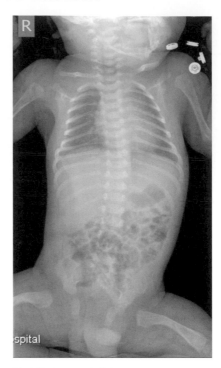

C: AP chest and abdomen

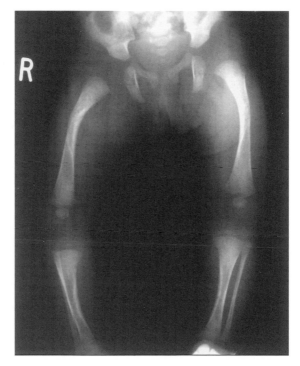

D: AP lower limbs

9.6 METABOLIC BONE DISEASE

- ➡ Osteopenia.
- ➡ Coarse trabeculae.
- ➡ Metaphyseal cupping, fraying and irregularity.
- ➡ Blood biochemistry:
  - ▶ serum calcium
  - ▶ serum phosphate.
- ➡ Dense metaphyseal lines with healing.

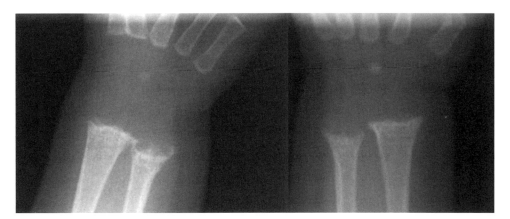

A: DP wrists

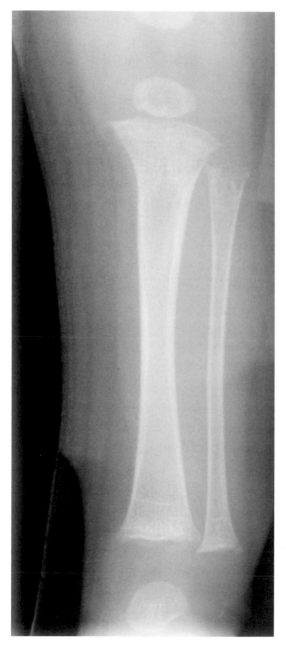

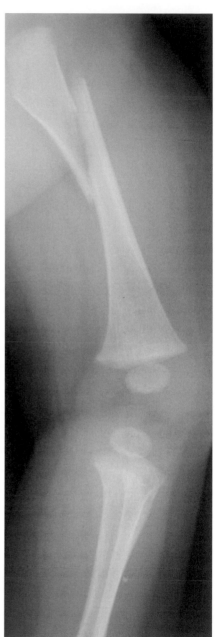

B: AP left tibia and fibula

C: Lateral left femur

9.7 OSTEOPATHY OF PREMATURITY

→ History of prematurity (note chronic lung changes in Figure A – this infant also had necrotising enterocolitis).
→ Generalised severe osteopenia.
→ Metaphyseal irregularity.
→ Coarse trabeculae.
→ Multiple fractures.

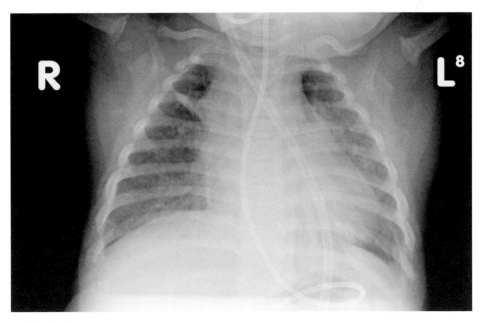

A: AP chest

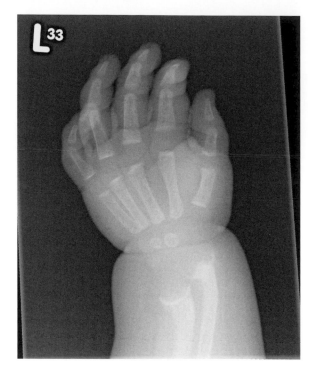

B: AP left arm

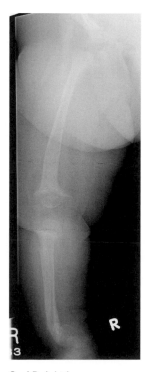

C: AP right leg

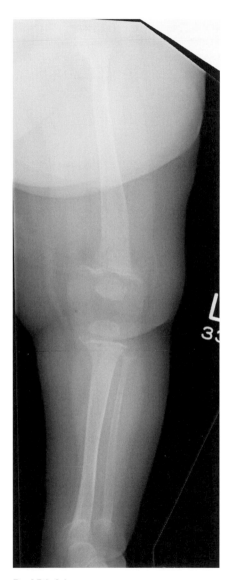

D: AP left leg

9.8 SCURVY

➡ Osteopenia.
➡ Wimberger's sign – the 'pencil' outline (dashed arrow).
➡ Pelcan spur (solid arrow).
➡ Calcified subperiosteal haemorrhage (arrow head).

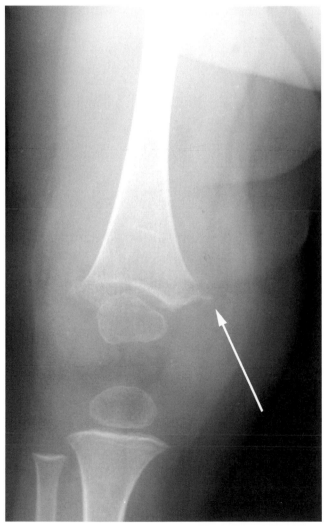

A: AP Right knee

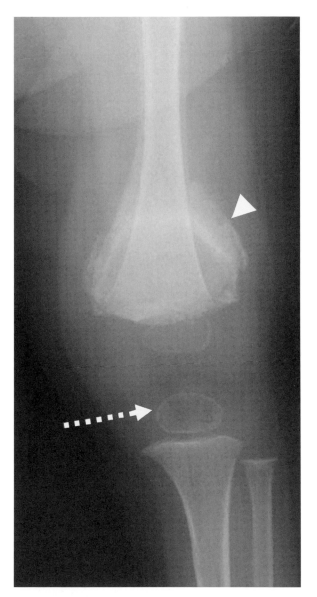

B: AP Left knee

9.9 SEPTIC ARTHRITIS

➡ Infection may be mistaken for abuse.
➡ CML (arrow) but also septic arthritis of the knee.
➡ It is rare for fractures in infants/children to become secondarily infected.
➡ The radiographs shown are of an infant who died of overwhelming sepsis.
  A subsequent sibling presented with multiple fractures typical of abuse.
➡ Note the intraosseous needle (broken arrow).

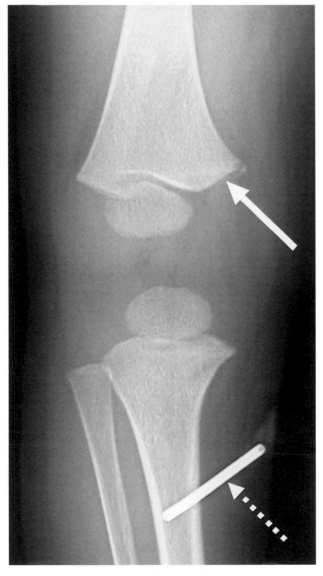

A: Post-mortem specimen radiograph, right knee

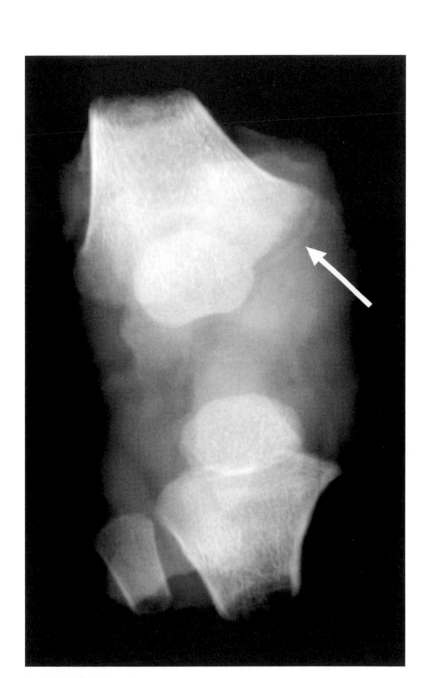

B: AP Right knee

9.10 OSTEOMYELITIS

➡ In this infant, the apparent CML (A) subsequently developed into full-blown osteomyelitis (B).

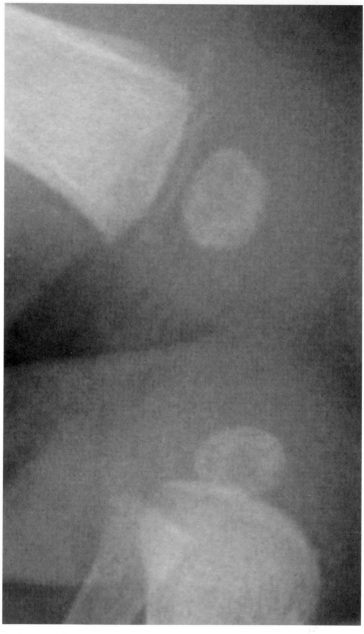

A: Lateral left femur

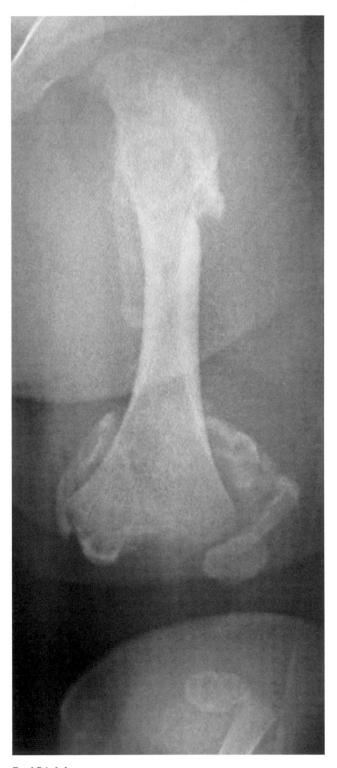

B: AP left femur

9.11 SKELETAL DYSPLASIAS WITH METAPHYSEAL INVOLVEMENT

➥ Symmetrical involvement of metaphyses with no change in radiographic appearance over 2–4 weeks:
  ◗ metaphyseal fractures resembling the CML of physical abuse
  ◗ metaphyseal cupping and irregularity.
➥ Platyspondyly.

A: Spondyloepimetaphyseal dysplasia, type Strudwick.
B: Spondylometaphyseal dysplasia, type Sutcliffe.

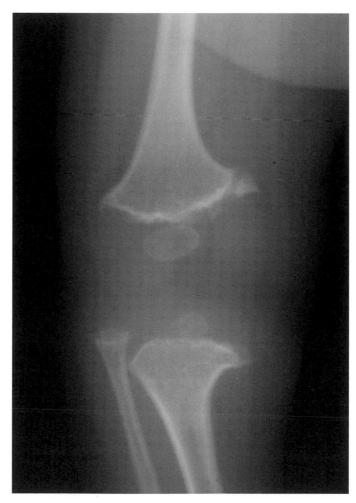

A: AP right knee

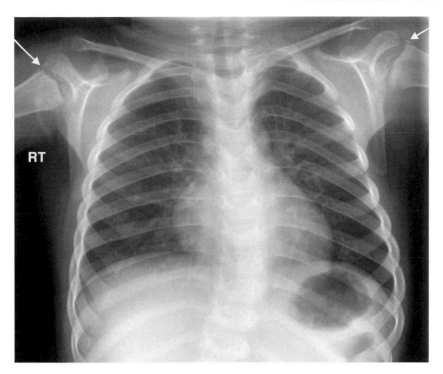

B1: AP chest

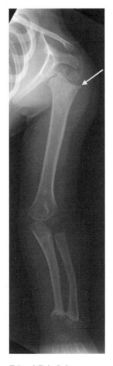

B2: AP left humerus

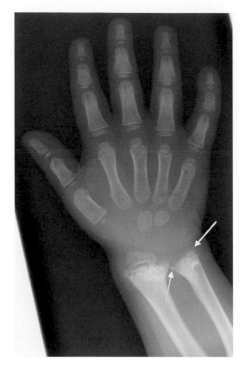

B3: DP right hand

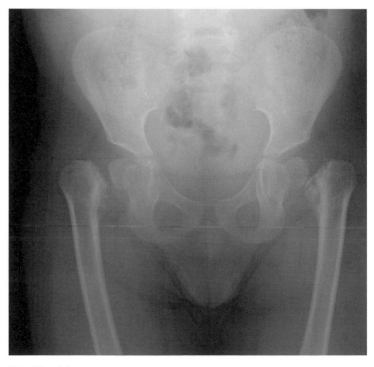

B4: AP pelvis

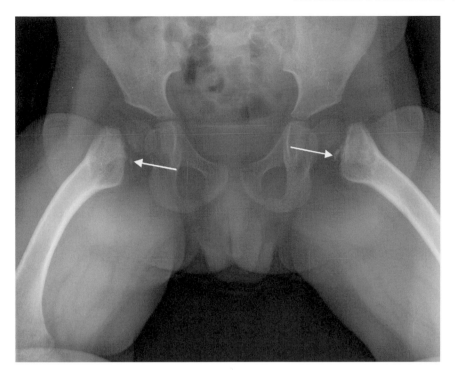

B5: Frog lateral pelvis

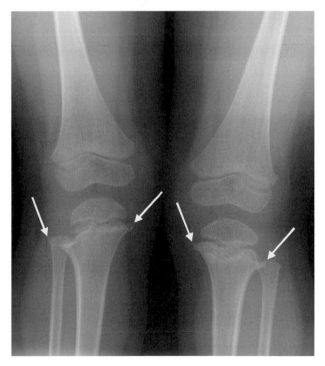

B6: AP right knee

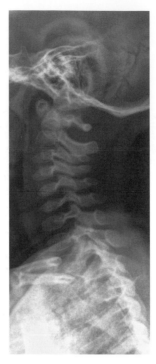

B8: Lateral cervical spine

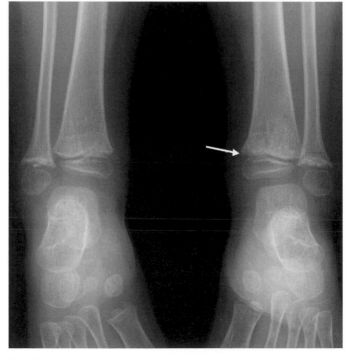

B7: AP ankles

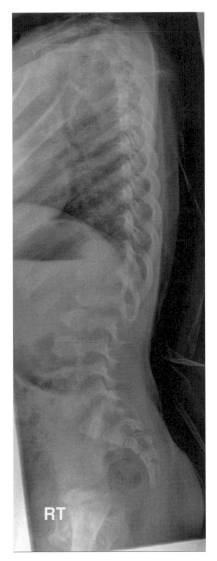

B9: Lateral thoracolumbar spine

CHAPTER 10

Fracture healing

There follow selected cases to illustrate the appearance of fractures at various stages of healing.

10.1 HUMERUS: FRACTURE SEPARATION THROUGH PROXIMAL GROWTH PLATE

➥ A: Day of presentation.
➥ B: Day 8.
➥ C: Day 56.
➥ D: Day 63.

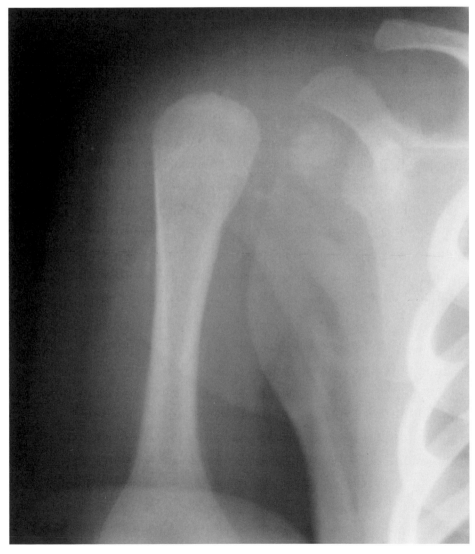

A

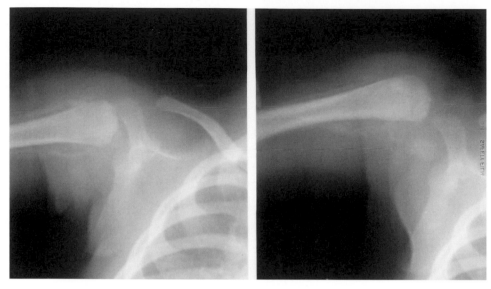

B

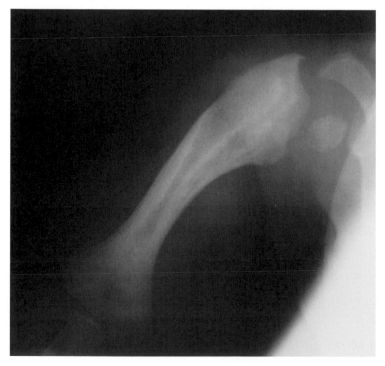

C

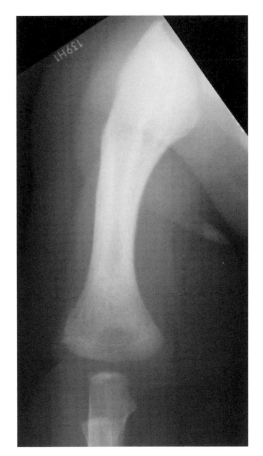

D

10.2 HUMERUS: TRANSVERSE MID SHAFT FRACTURE

➡ A: Day of presentation.
➡ B: Day 5.
➡ C: Day 26.

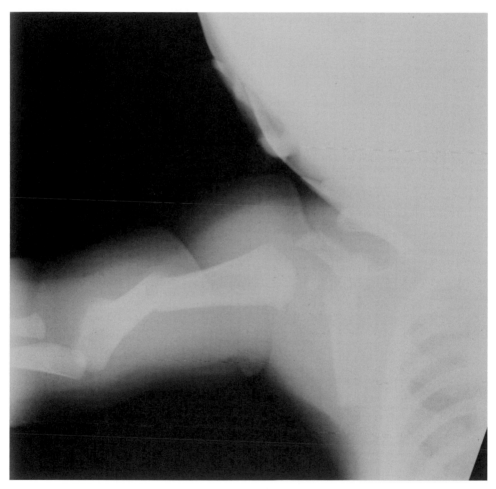

A

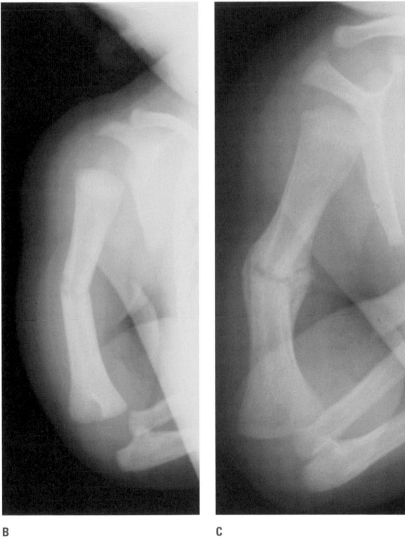

B

C

10.3 HUMERUS: OBLIQUE MID SHAFT FRACTURE

➡ A: Day of presentation.
➡ B: Day 4.
➡ C: Day 11.
➡ D: Day 18.
➡ E: Day 32.

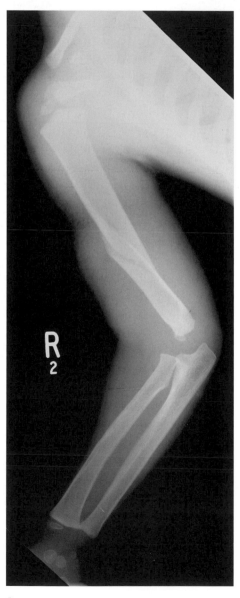

A

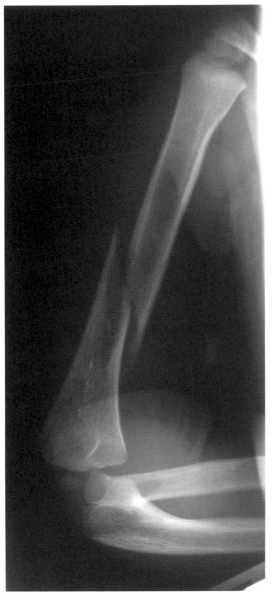

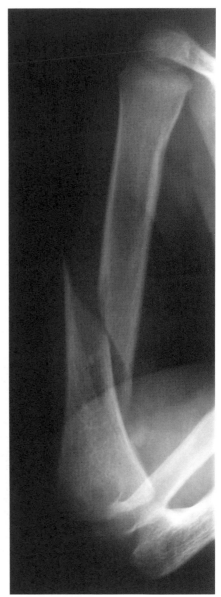

B

C

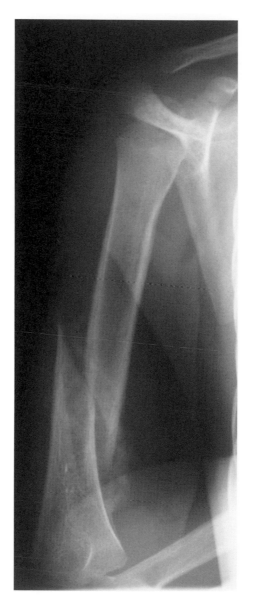

D

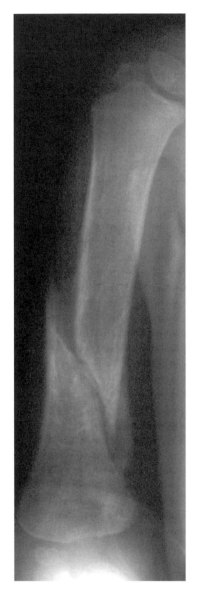

E

10.4 HUMERUS: ANGULATED MID SHAFT FRACTURE

➥ A: Day of presentation.
  ▶ Acute humeral fracture, healing ulna fracture.
➥ B: Day 3.
  ▶ Skeletal survey revealed multiple healing rib fractures.
➥ C: 3 months and 3 weeks after presentation.

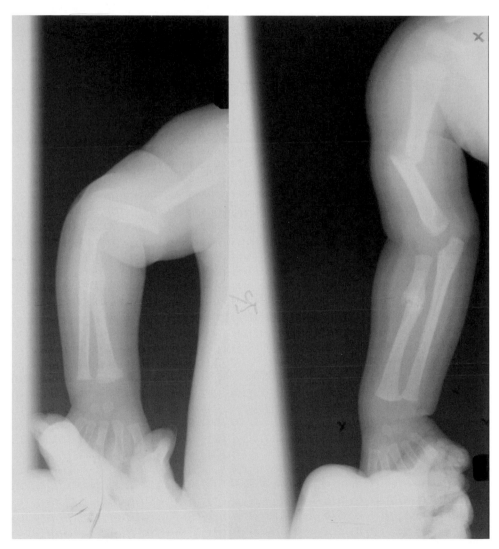

A

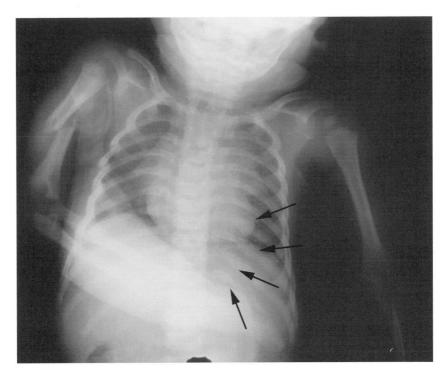

B

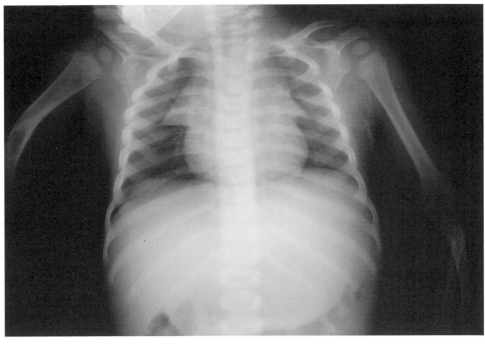

C

10.5 HUMERUS: TRANSVERSE DISTAL SHAFT FRACTURE

➥ Infant aged three months at presentation.
➥ A: Day of presentation.
➥ B: Day 9.

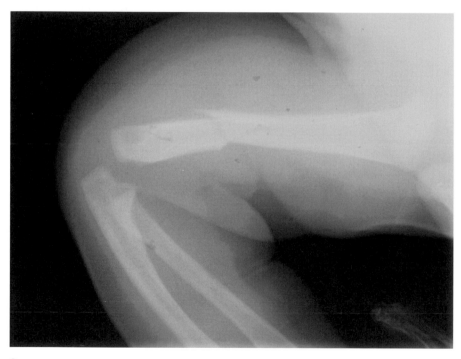

A

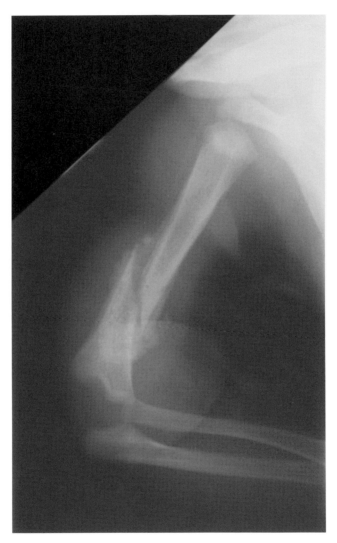

B

10.6 HUMERUS: SUPRACONDYLAR FRACTURE

➡ A: Day of presentation.
➡ B: Day 75.
➡ Notice also the proximal metaphyseal fracture.

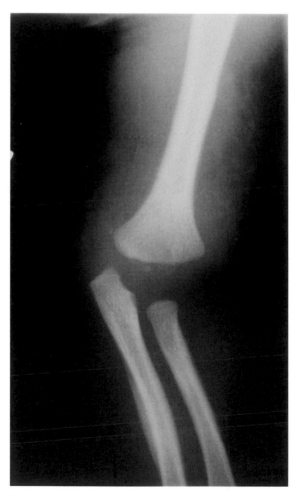

A

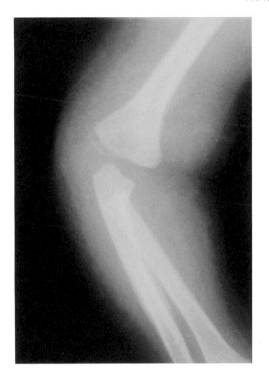

A

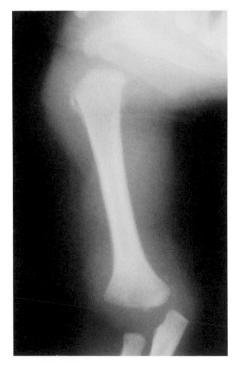

B

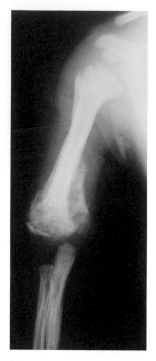

C

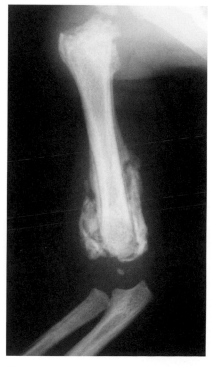

C

10.7 HUMERUS: SUPRACONDYLAR FRACTURE

➥ A: Day of presentation.
➥ B: Day 5.
➥ C: Day 53.

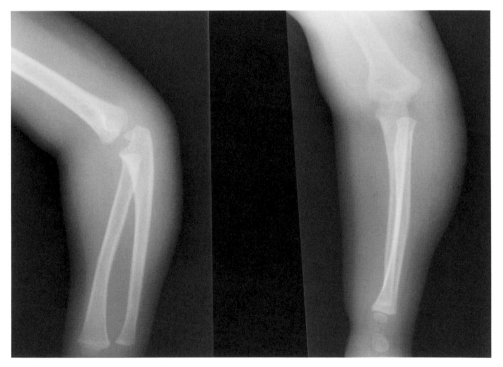

A

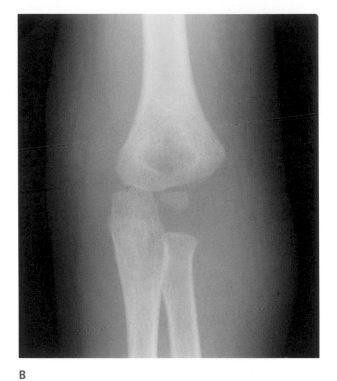

B

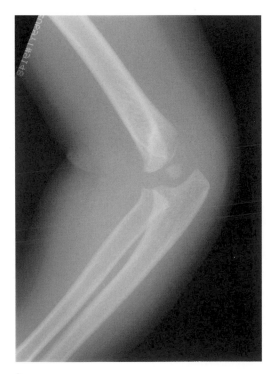

B

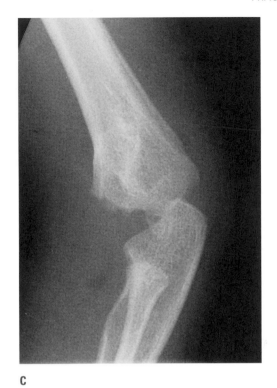

C

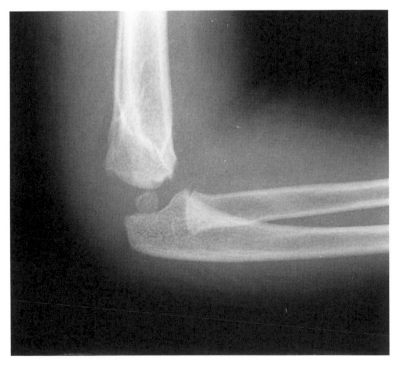

C

10.8 HUMERUS: SUPRACONDYLAR FRACTURE

➡ A: Day of presentation.
➡ B: Day 5.
➡ C: Day 53.

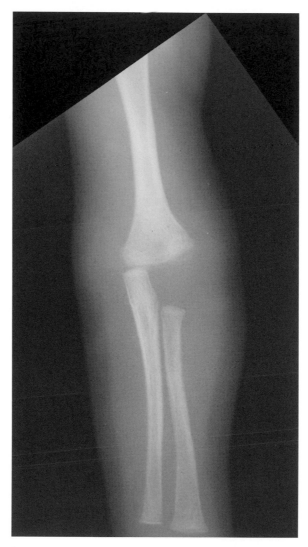

A

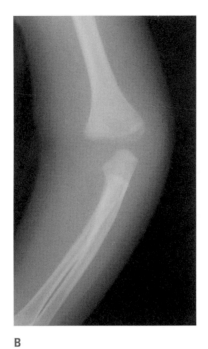

B

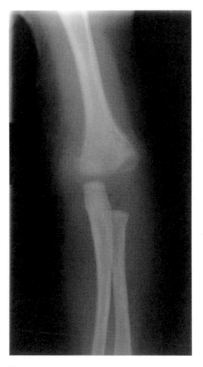

B

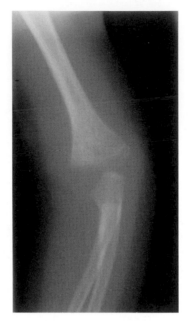

B

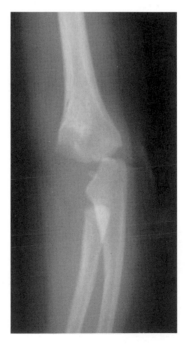

C

10.9 RADIUS AND ULNA: ANGULATED TRANSVERSE FRACTURES

➡ A: Day 10.
➡ B: Day 47.

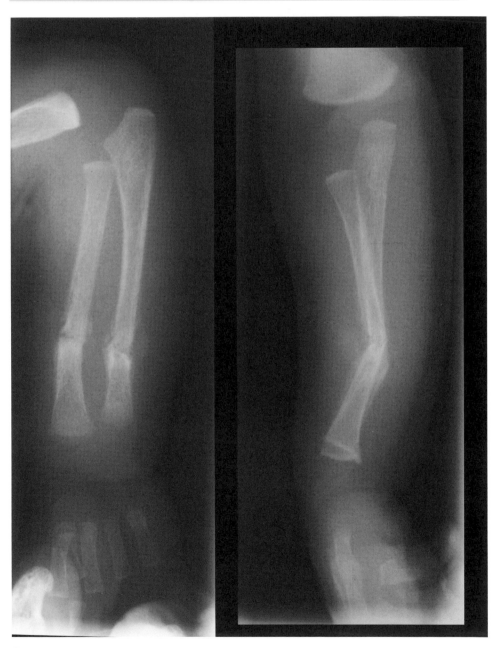

A

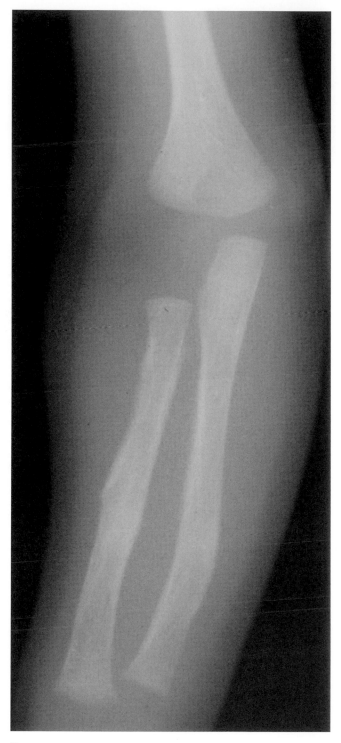

B

10.10 FEMUR: BILATERAL NECK FRACTURES

➥ Child aged 13.5 months at presentation.
➥ A: Day of presentation.
➥ B: Day 3
➥ C: Day 17.

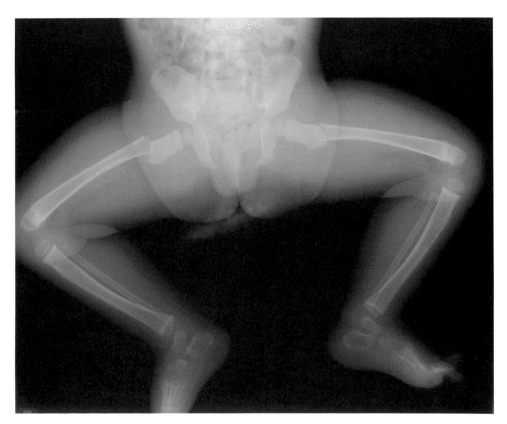

A

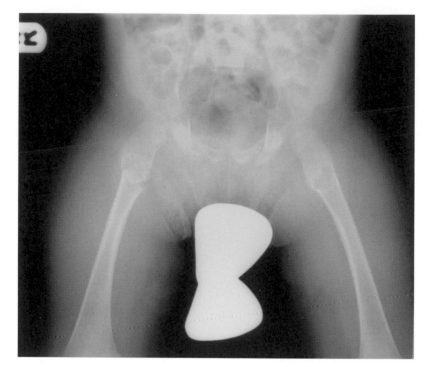

B

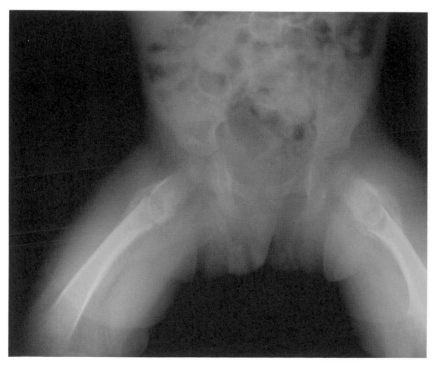

C

10.11 FEMUR: UNDISPLACED MID SHAFT SPIRAL FRACTURE

➥ A: Day of presentation.
➥ B: Day 2.
➥ C: Day 9.
➥ D: Day 16.

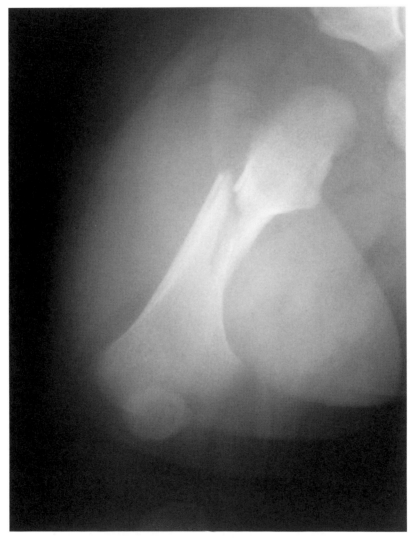

A

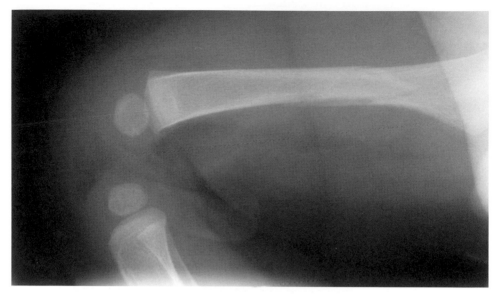

B

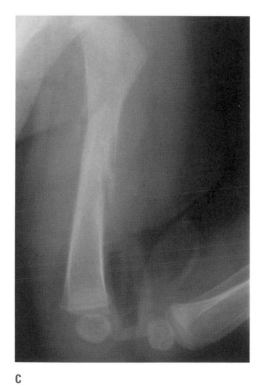

C

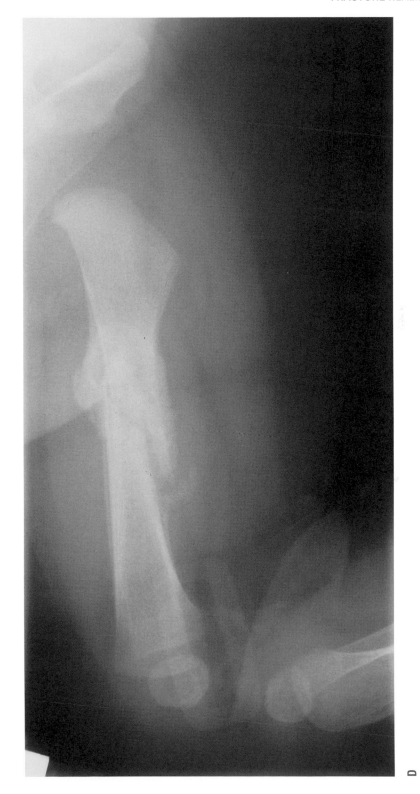

D

10.12 FEMUR: MINIMALLY DISPLACED MID SHAFT SPIRAL FRACTURE

➡ A: Day of presentation.
➡ B: Day 13.
➡ C: Day 27.

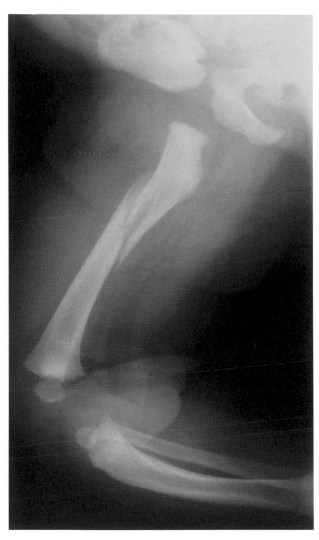

A

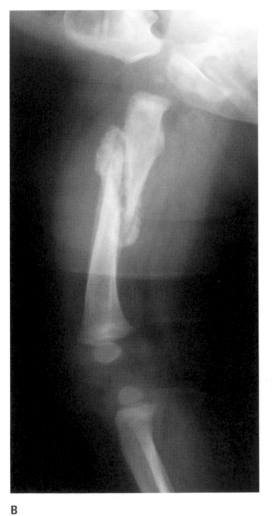

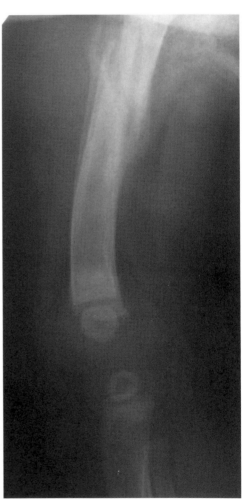

B

C

10.13 FEMUR: DISPLACED ANGULATED MID SHAFT SPIRAL FRACTURE

➥ A: Day of presentation.
➥ B: Day 10.
➥ C: Day 15.
➥ D: Day 46.
➥ E: 16 months.

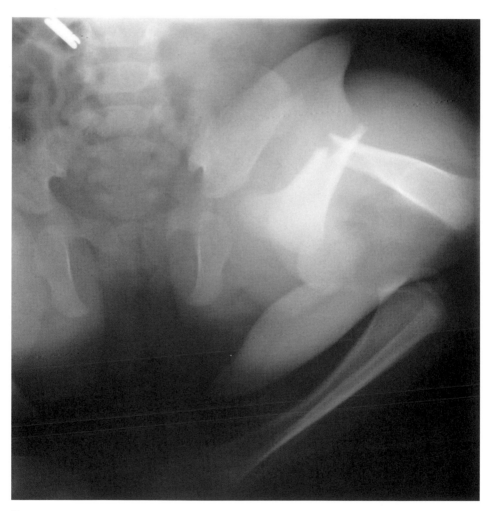

A

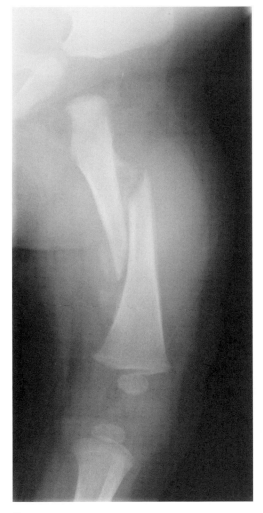

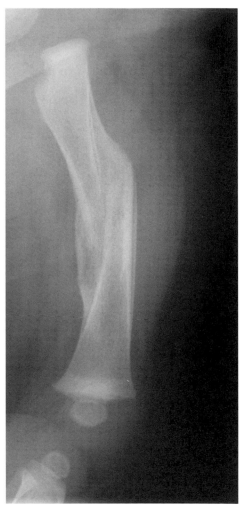

B

C

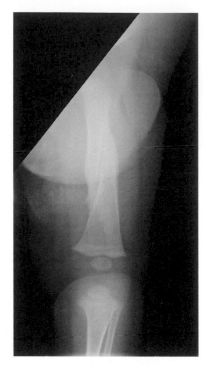

D

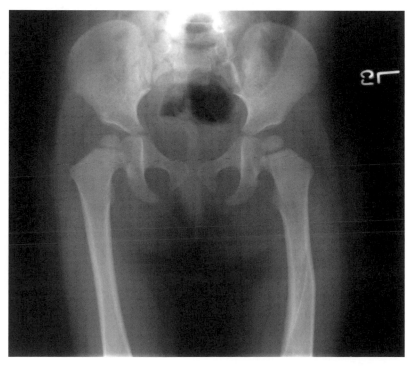

E

10.14 FEMUR: DISPLACED TRANSVERSE FRACTURE MID SHAFT

➥ A: Day of presentation.
➥ B: Day 1.
➥ C: Day 6.
➥ D: Day 14.
➥ E: Day 28.

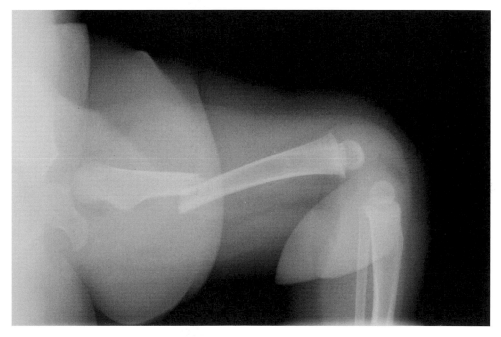

A

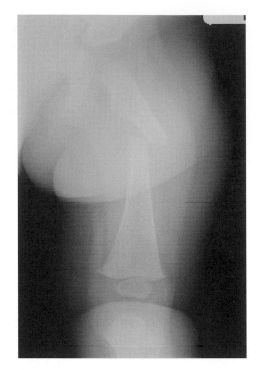

A

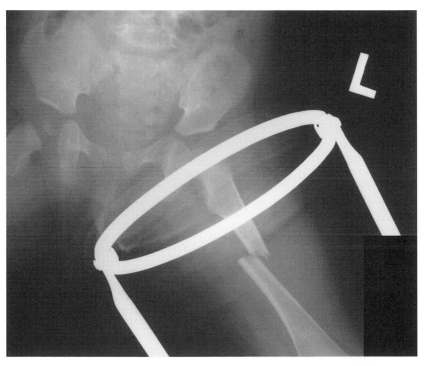

B

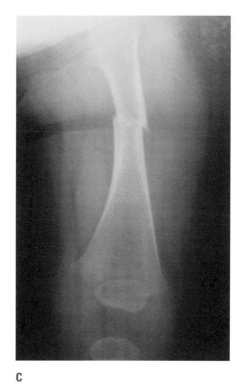

C

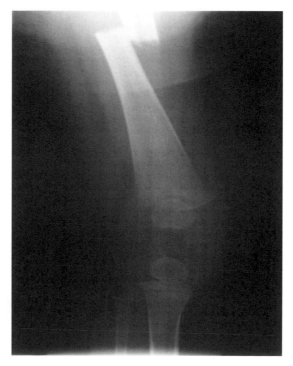

C

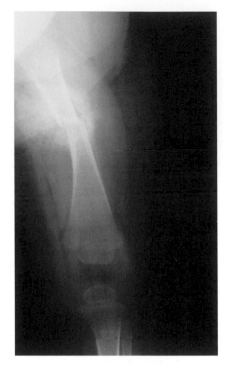

D

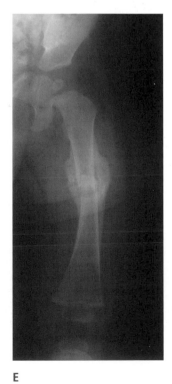

E

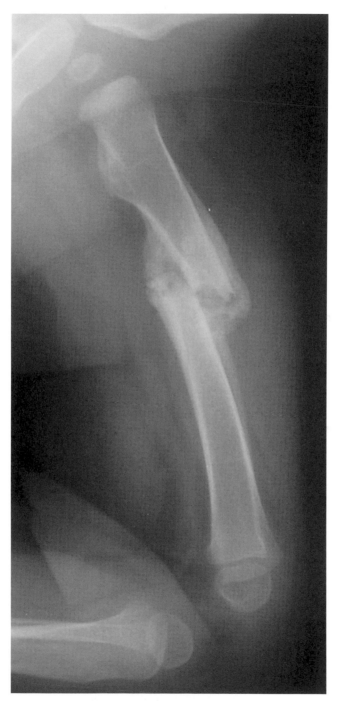

E

10.15 FEMUR: DISPLACED TRANSVERSE FRACTURE DISTAL SHAFT

➥ A: Day of presentation.
➥ B: Day 1.
➥ C: Day 14.

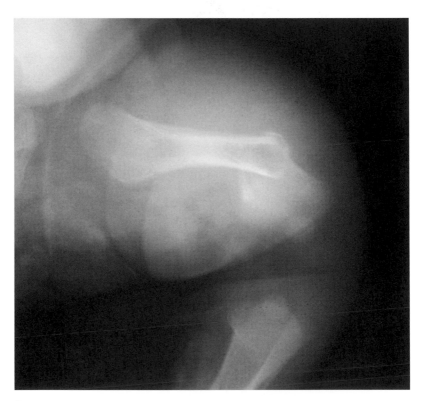

A

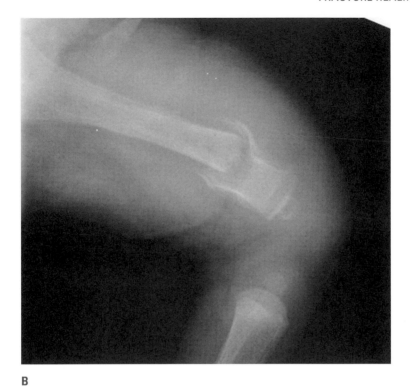

B

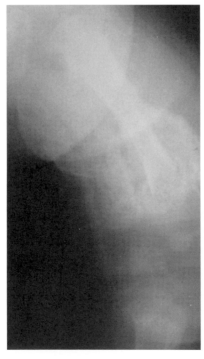

C

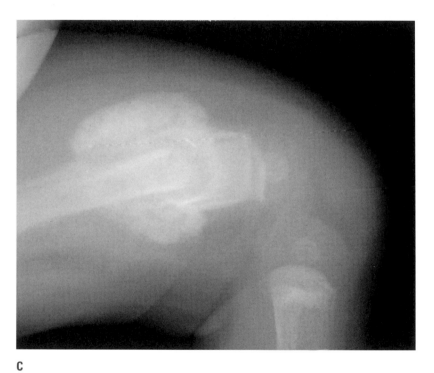

C

10.16 FEMUR: IMPACTED FRACTURE DISTAL SHAFT

➥ A: Day of presentation.
➥ B: 4 months.

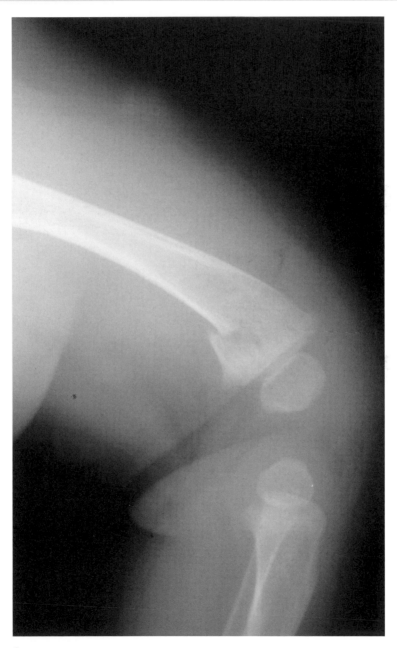

A

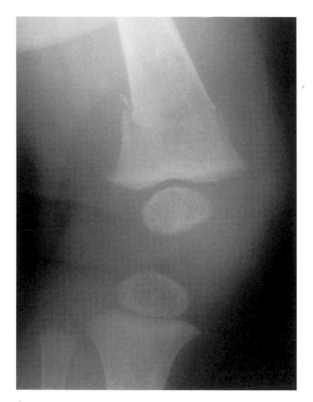

A

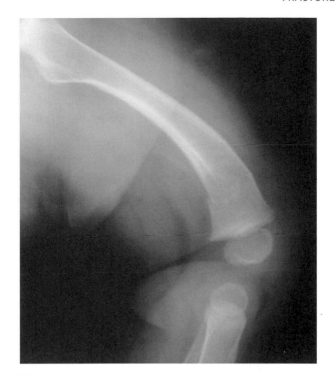

B

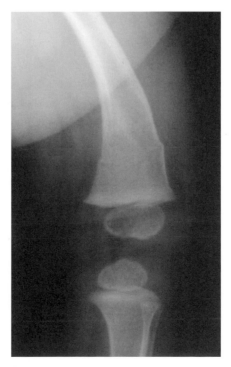

B

10.17 TIBIA: PROXIMAL CML

➥ A: Day of presentation.
➥ B: Day 32.

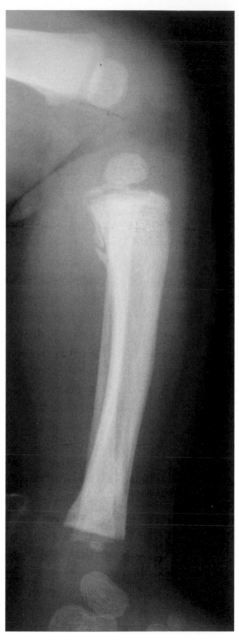

A

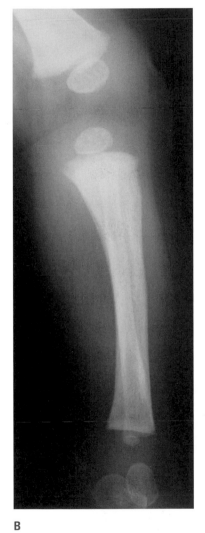

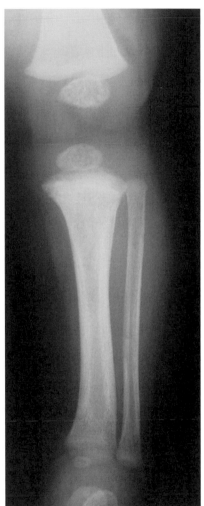

B

B

10.18 TIBIA: ANGULATED SPIRAL FRACTURE

➥ Infant aged 33 days at presentation.
➥ A, B: Day of presentation.
➥ C: Day 20.

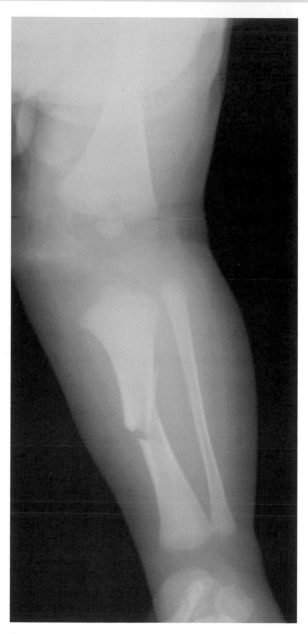

A

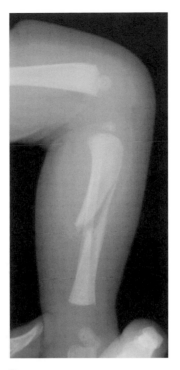

B

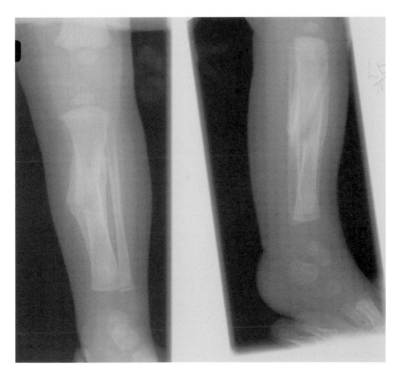

C

10.19 TIBIA: OBLIQUE FRACTURE DISTAL SHAFT

➥ A: Day of presentation.
  ▶ Note fracture line through callus indicating repetitive trauma (*see* Plate 5.4)
➥ B: Day 23.
➥ C: 4 months.

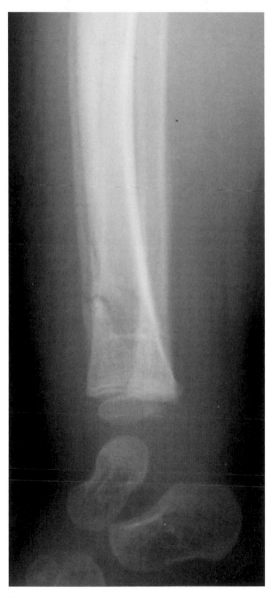

A

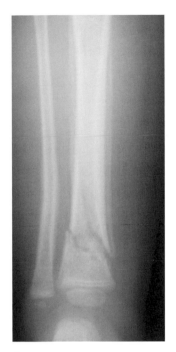

A

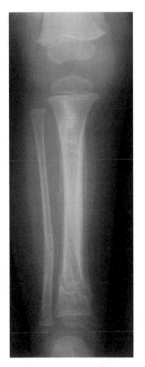

B

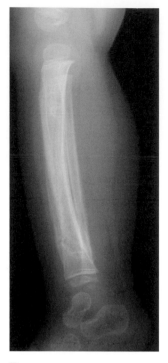

B

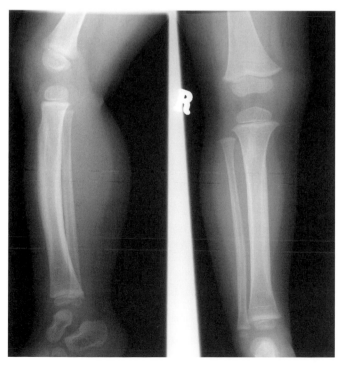

C

10.20 MULTIPLE RIB FRACTURES

➡ A: Bone scan on day of presentation.
➡ B: 5 days after bone scan.
➡ C: 17 days after bone scan.

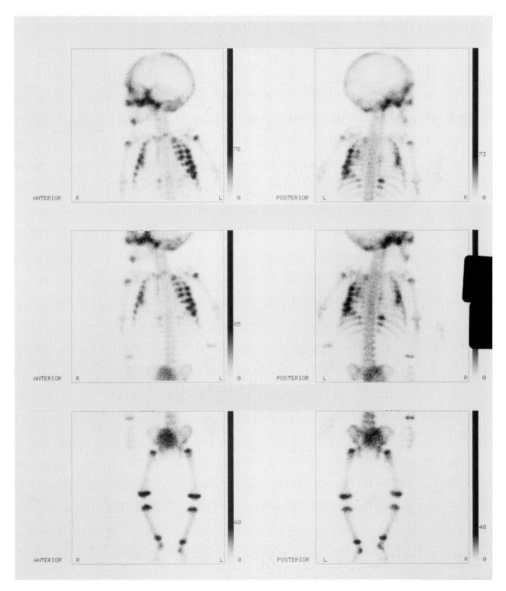

A

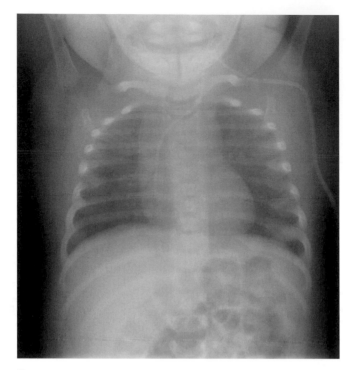

B

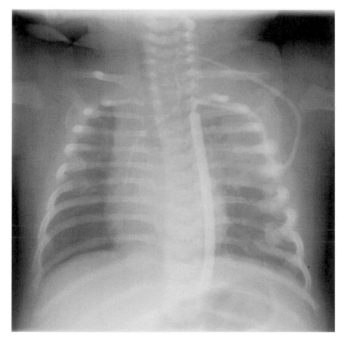

C

10.21 MULTIPLE RIB FRACTURES

- ➡ A: Day of presentation with respiratory symptoms.
- ➡ B: Day 27 – acute forearm fracture, therefore skeletal survey repeated.
- ➡ C: Day 28 (after original presentation).
  - ❯ In retrospect, healing fractures of the posterior ends of the left 6th and 7th (and possibly 5th) ribs are visible on the initial radiograph (D).

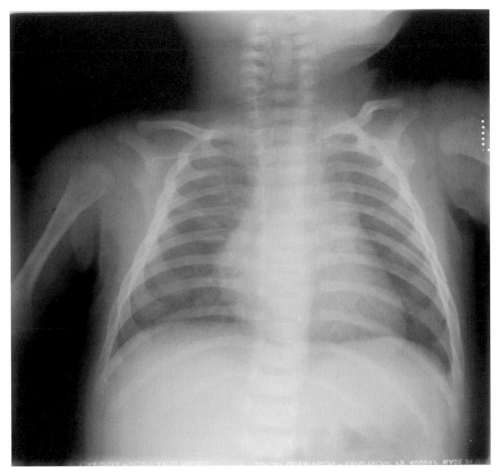

A

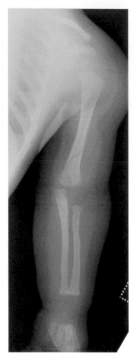

B

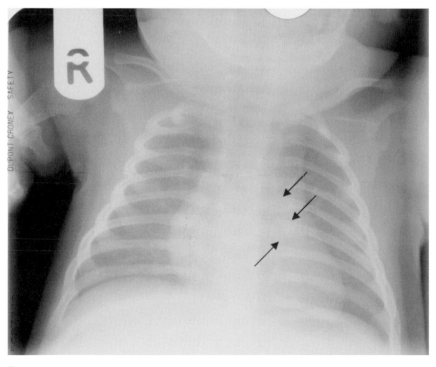

C

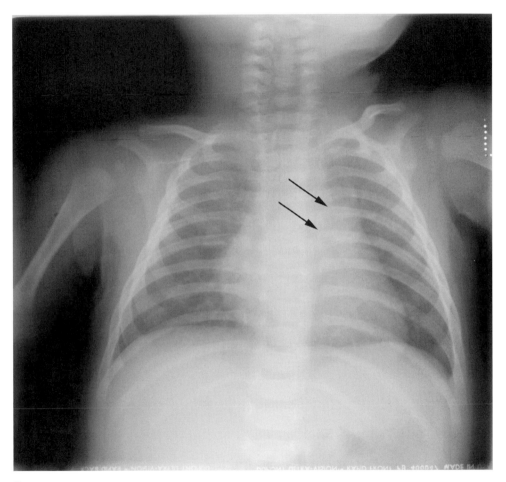

D

10.22 MULTIPLE RIB FRACTURES

➥ A: Day of presentation with respiratory distress – fractures <7–10 days.
➥ B: Day 14.
➥ C: Day 43.

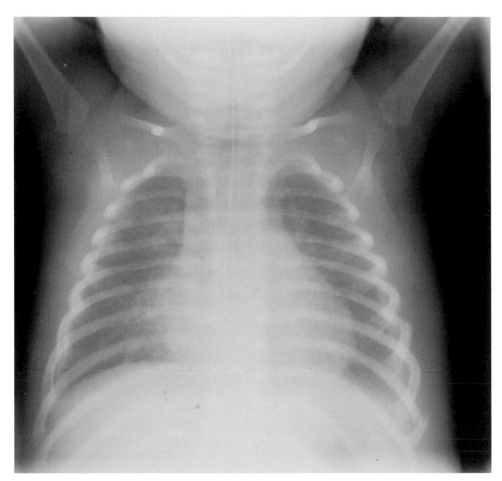

A

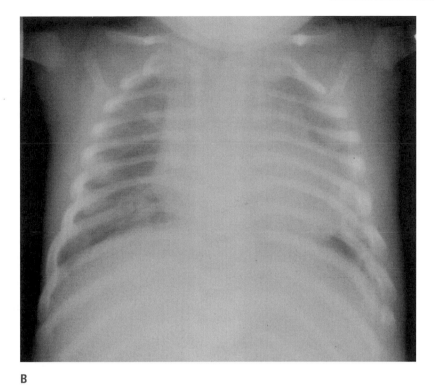

B

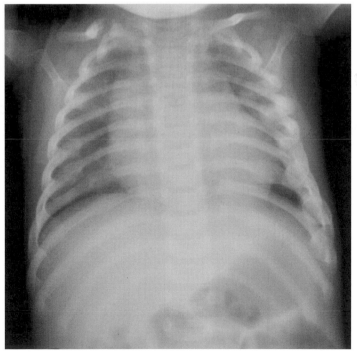

C

10.23 MULTIPLE RIB FRACTURES

➥ A: Day of presentation.
➥ B: 4 weeks.
➥ C: 6 months.

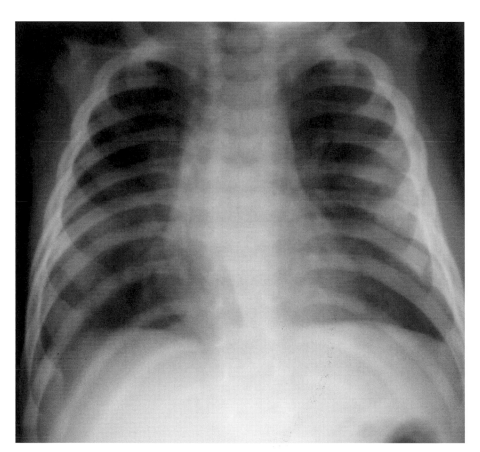

A

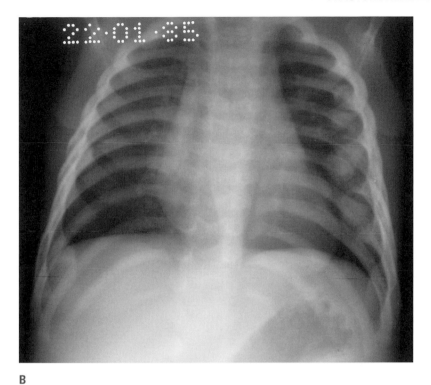

B

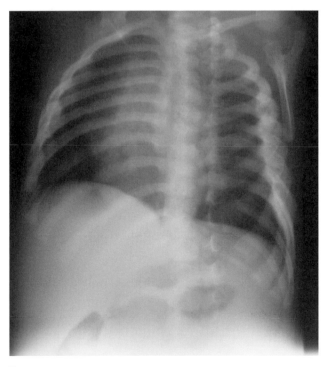

B

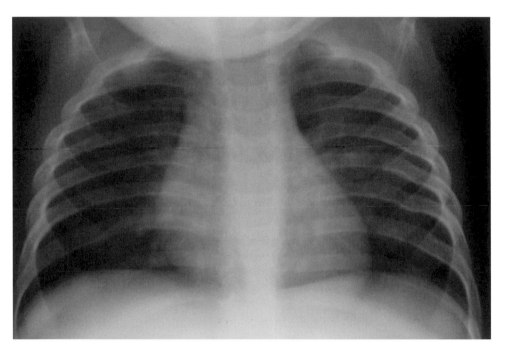

C

The following are selected cases to illustrate the different presentations and common dilemmas faced by radiologists working in the field of child protection.

We make no apologies for the quality of some of the images/surveys; they remain as we received them.

Historical details have been altered where we have thought it necessary, in order to maintain anonymity.

CHAPTER 11

Cases

CASE 1A

History:
- a 12-month-old infant presented with an acute abdomen.

Past medical history:
- three weeks previously she had been seen in A&E
- at that time her mother fell down a flight of stairs while carrying her
- the infant was said to have hit her head on concrete
- no loss of consciousness or other associated symptoms
- clinical examination revealed right forehead contusion and superficial abrasion
- otherwise normal with a GCS of 15
- a skull radiograph was **not** performed at this time
- she was discharged following head injury advice
- no other past medical or family history of note.

Initial radiographs:
- what are the findings?
- how should this infant be managed?

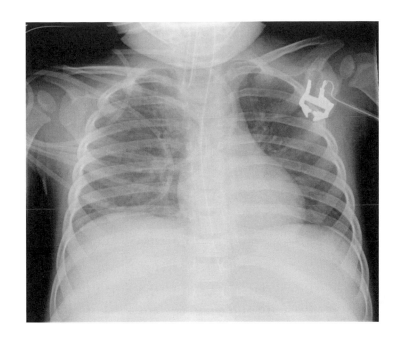

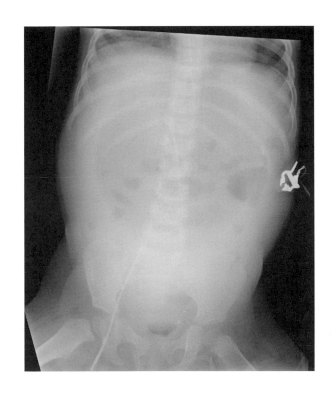

CASE 1B

➡ There are fractures of the right posterior 10th and 11th ribs.
  ▶ The callus is mature but the fracture lines remain visible.
  ▶ These fractures are 4–6 weeks old.
➡ There is evidence of free intraperitoneal air; 'football' sign.
  ▶ Duodenal perforation was found at surgery.
➡ Once the infant is stabilised a skeletal survey should be performed.

Skeletal survey:
➡ date any other injuries identified
➡ is the history of a fall three weeks earlier of any relevance?

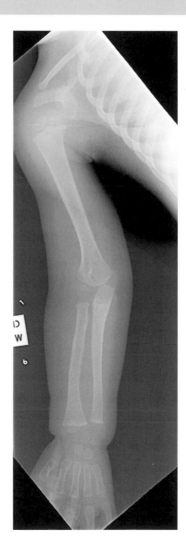

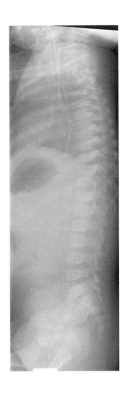

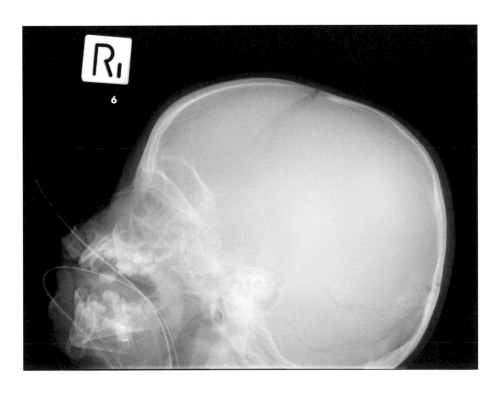

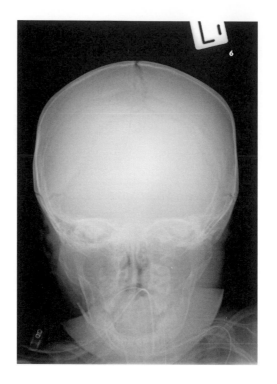

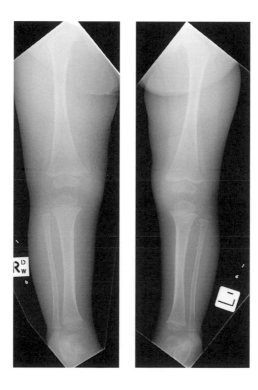

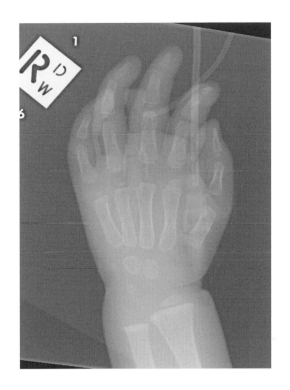

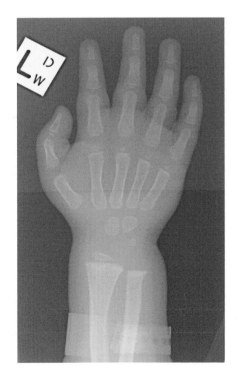

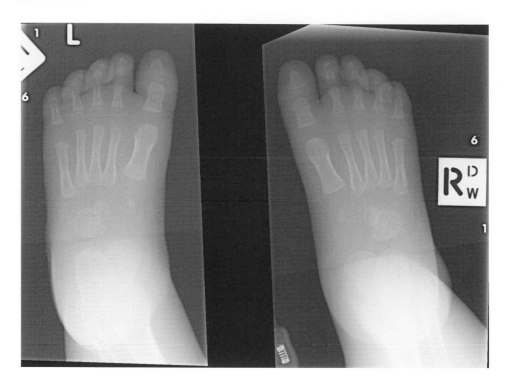

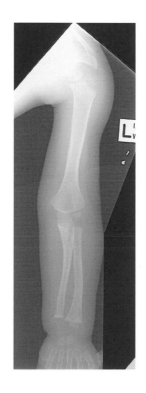

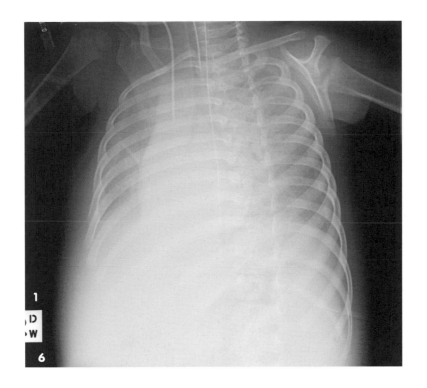

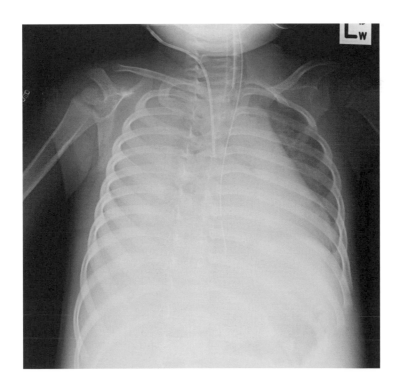

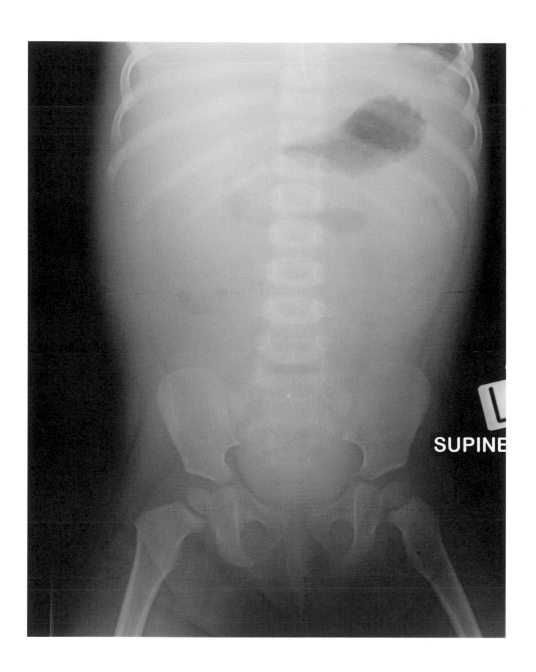

CASE 1C

➡ There is a fracture of the left occipital bone.
  ▶ There is no associated soft tissue swelling; therefore this fracture is greater than 10 days old.
➡ Although the timing is appropriate, this infant's occipital skull fracture is highly unlikely to have arisen from a fall onto her forehead.

Comment:
➡ should she have had skull radiographs on initial presentation?
  ▶ should skull radiographs routinely be performed in all infants with head injury?

CASE 2A

History:
- a 15-day-old infant with swelling of the left femur
  - uncomplicated spontaneous vaginal delivery
- her father stated that he had leant over her leg while trying to retrieve a feeding bottle.

Skeletal survey:
- date any injuries identified.

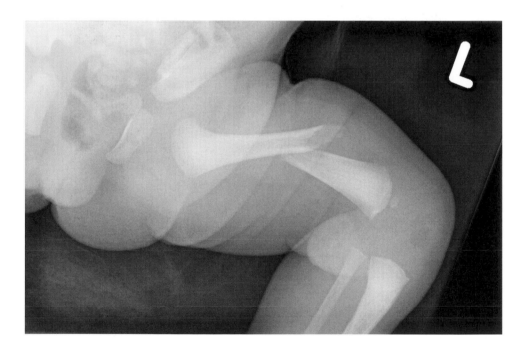

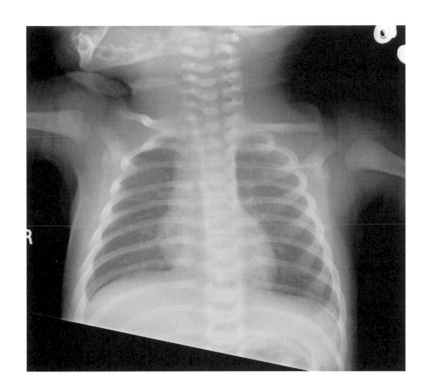

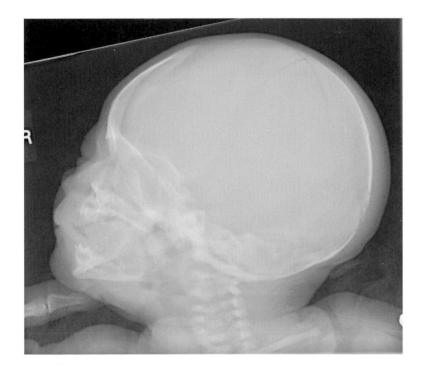

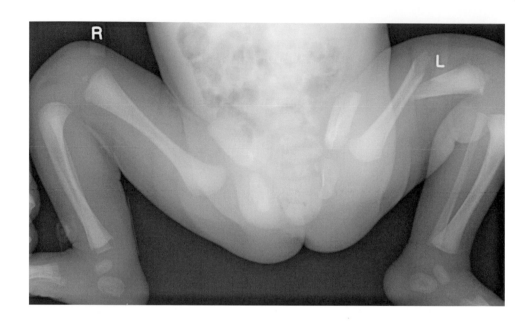

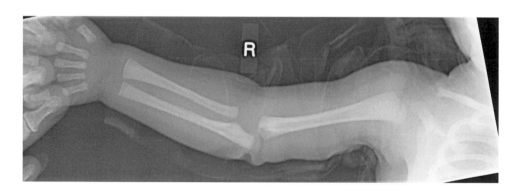

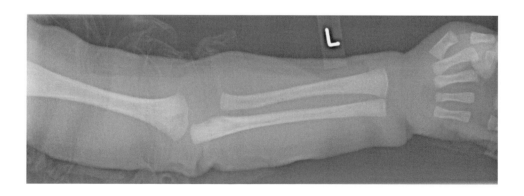

CASE 2B

➡ There are four fractures:
- ▶ short oblique fracture mid femoral shaft
  - — no periosteal reaction, so <7–10 days
  - — no soft tissue swelling, so probably <24 hours
- ▶ CML right distal tibia
  - — <4 weeks old
- ▶ CML right distal fibula
  - — <4 weeks old
- ▶ bilateral parietal skull fractures
  - — associated soft tissue swelling, best seen on CT scout, so at least one of these fractures is <7–10 days old.

➡ The skeletal survey was completed the following day.

Skeletal survey:

➡ comment on the femoral fracture.

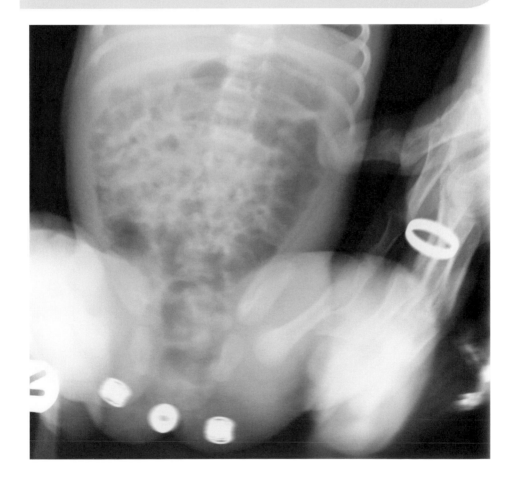

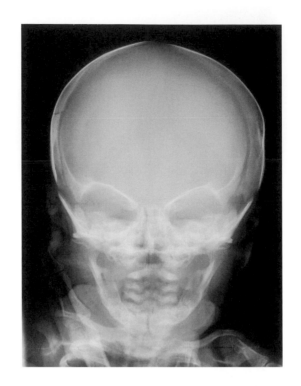

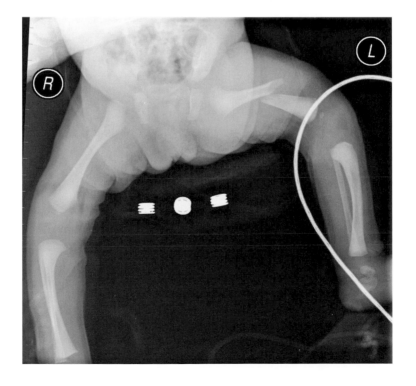

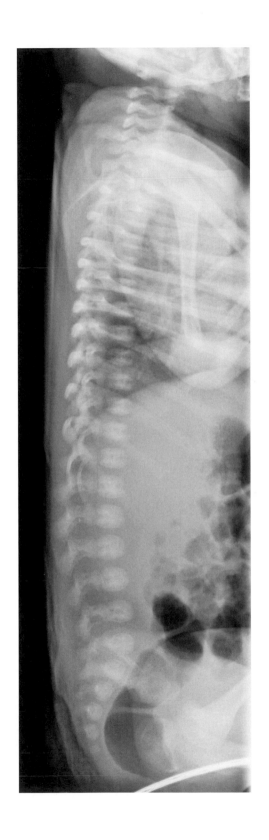

CASE 2C

➡ There is now some soft tissue swelling, supporting the initial suspicion that the femoral fracture was sustained on the day of presentation.

Serial radiographs:
➡ A: Day 7
➡ B: Day 14
➡ C: Day 21.

Discussion:
➡ the possibility was also raised of a left proximal tibial metaphyseal fracture. The following serial radiographs support this view.

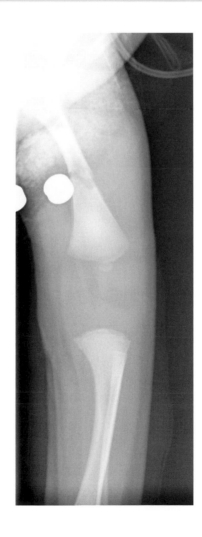

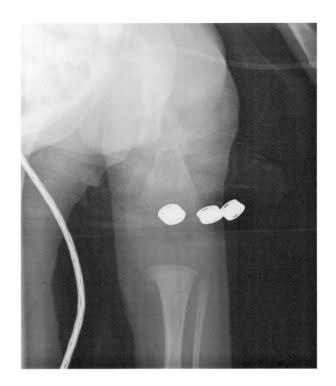

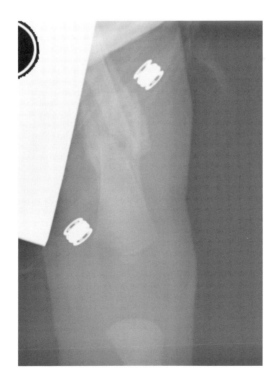

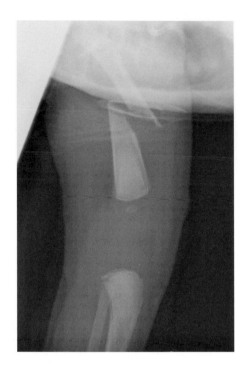

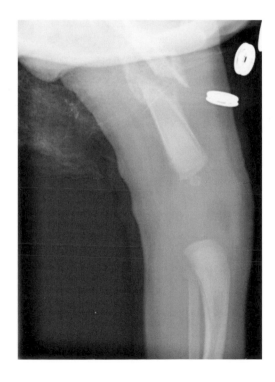

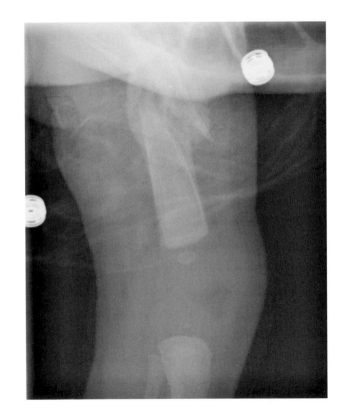

CASE 3A

History:
- ➡ this stillborn infant was the product of a concealed pregnancy
- ➡ after delivery she was accidentally dropped onto a carpeted floor
- ➡ mother hid her body, but she was discovered by other family members.

Skeletal survey:
- ➡ identify the injuries
- ➡ how is the history inconsistent with the radiological findings?

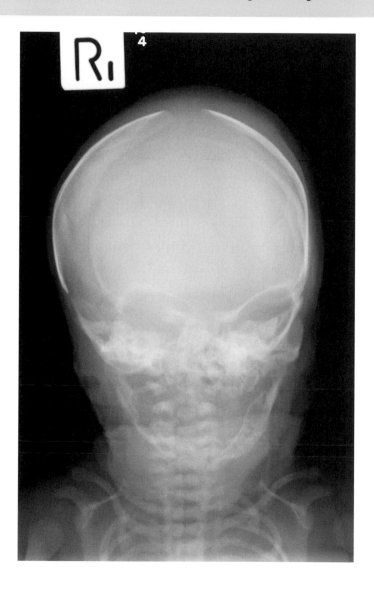

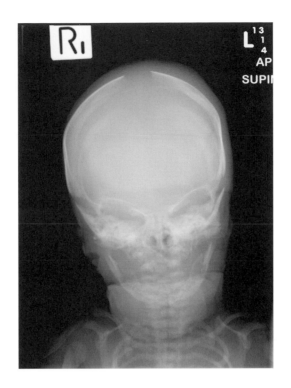

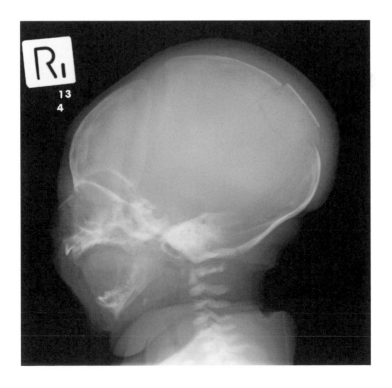

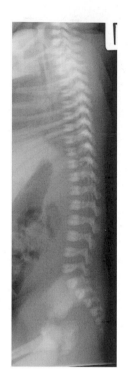

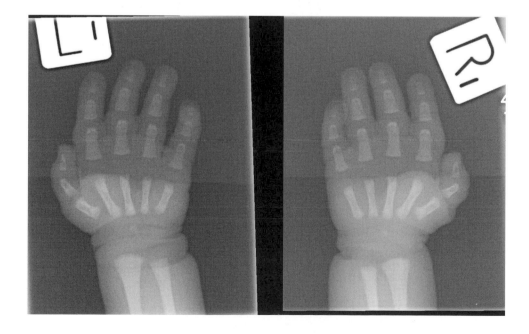

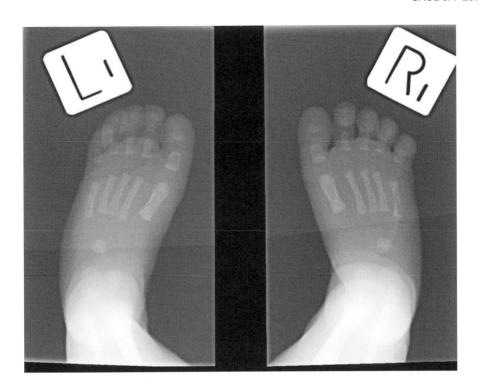

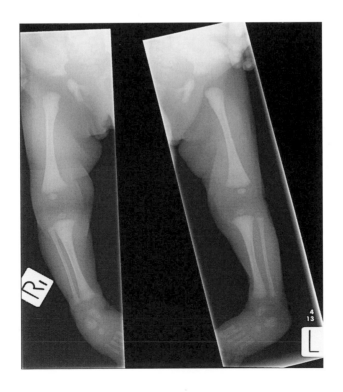

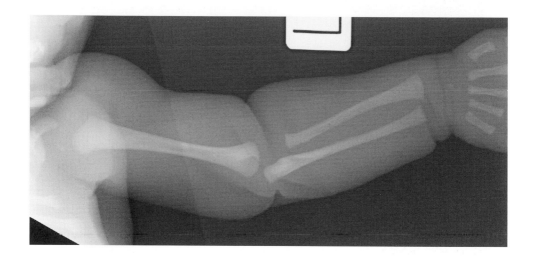

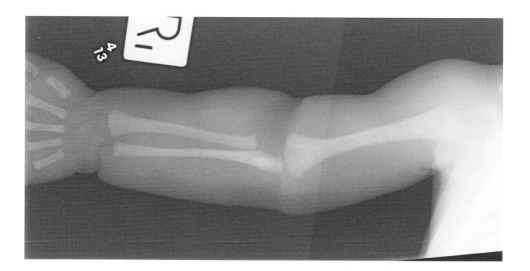

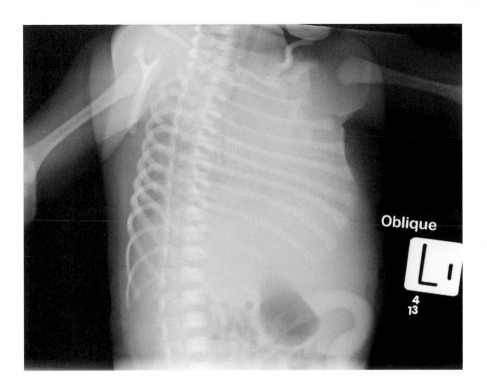

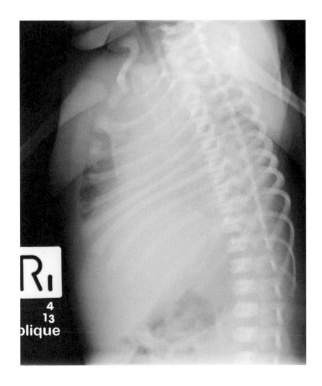

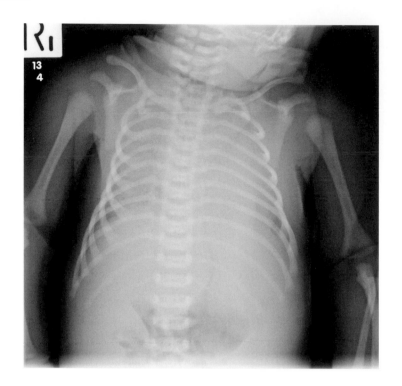

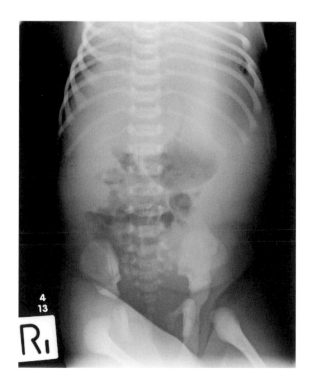

CASE 3B

➡ There is a complex parietal skull fracture with associated scalp swelling.
➡ Air in the lung bases, stomach and bowel suggest a live birth, thus escalating this from a case of concealed pregnancy to one of murder.

CASE 4A

History:
- a 16-month-old child brought to A&E after his father noticed he would not weight bear on his left leg
- the child was in the care of his father and stepmother. His mother lived elsewhere and had been diagnosed with a personality disorder
- the day before, the child had apparently fallen from approximately two feet onto a wooden floor, but did not appear to have suffered any harm.

Leg radiograph:
- what are your findings?

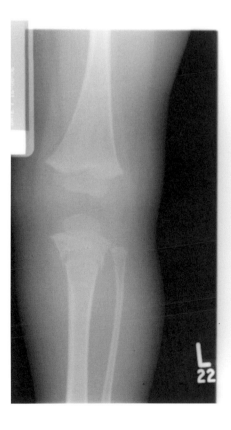
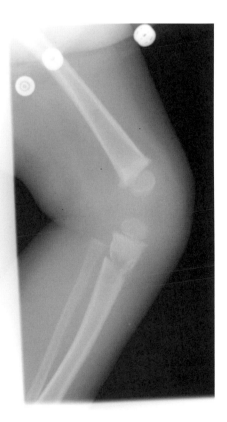

CASE 4B

➥ There is a transverse fracture of the proximal tibial metadiaphysis. There is associated soft tissue swelling.
➥ The local interpretation of the lateral radiograph was that there was a proximal tibial bone cyst, and that this therefore represented a pathological fracture.
➥ POP was applied, and the child returned home.

Follow up:
➥ subsequently, the child re-presented several times because the POP kept 'slipping'. Finally 'blue plaster' was applied
➥ three weeks following initial presentation, the child returned to A&E in extremis
➥ his father had found him unresponsive in his bed, with blood on the sheets and behind his left knee. The plaster was loose, and there was a deep horizontal laceration of the soft tissues of the left popliteal fossa
➥ a skeletal survey was performed prior to post-mortem histopathology.

Post-mortem skeletal survey:
➥ list the abnormalities
➥ any comments on the initial interpretation?

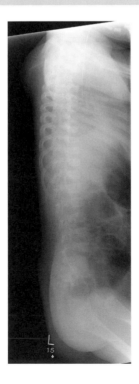

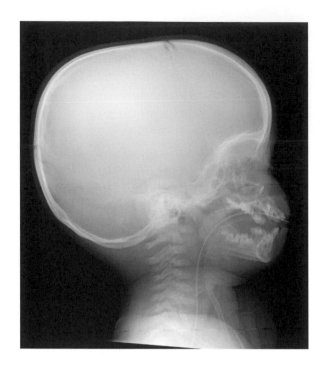

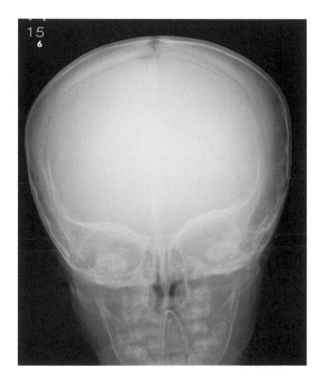

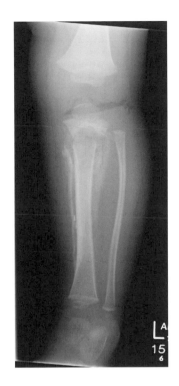

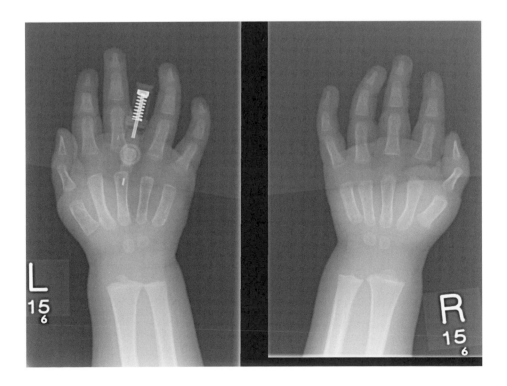

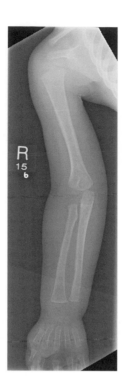

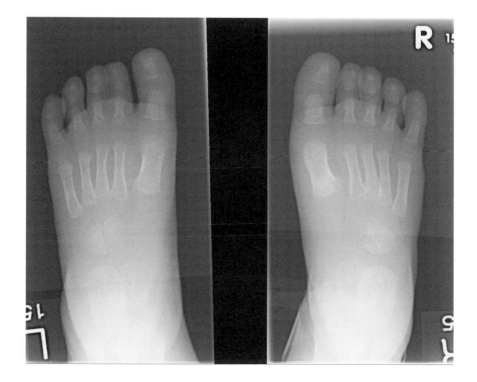

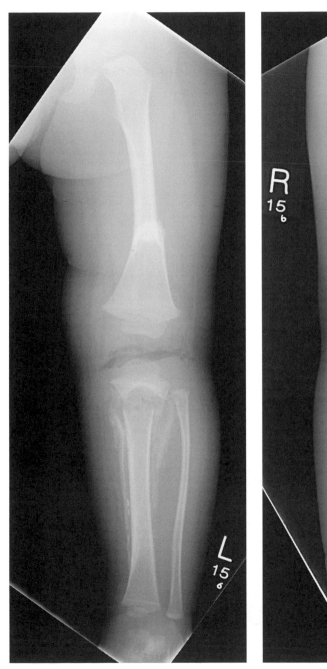
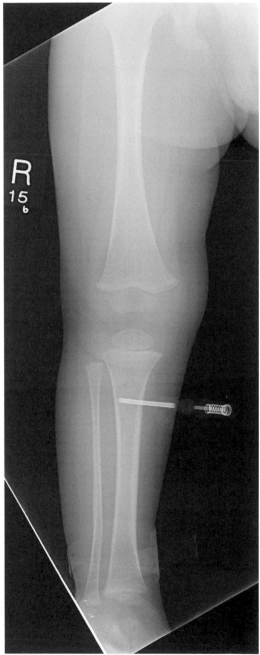

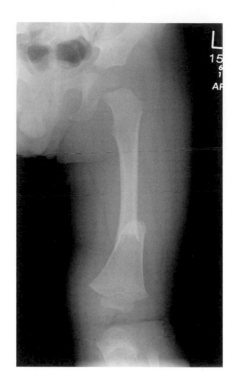

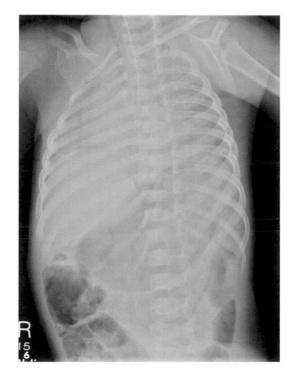

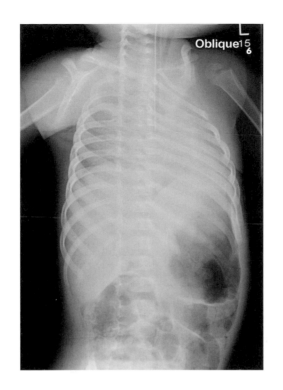

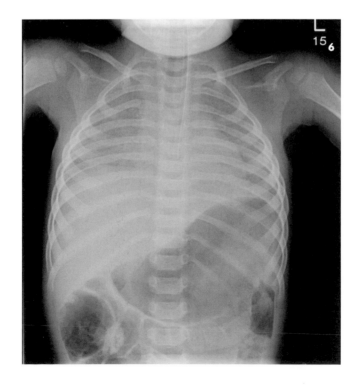

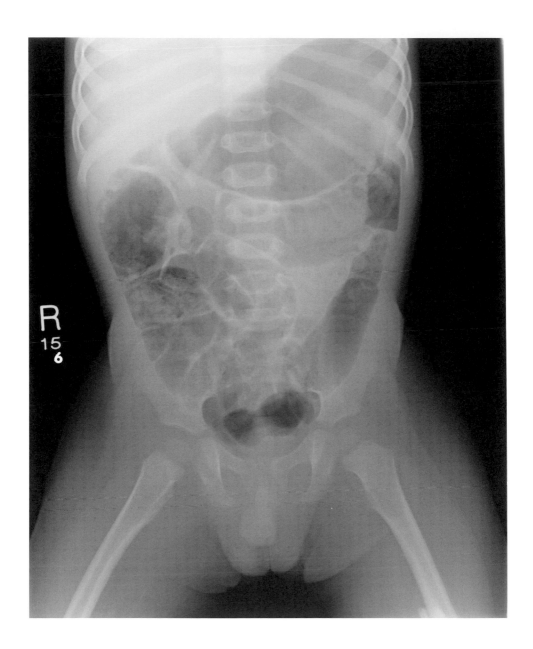

CASE 4C

➥ The following injuries are identified:
- ▶ transverse fracture left femur with very early periosteal reaction along the lateral edge of the proximal fragment – this fracture is 7–10 days of age
- ▶ metaphyseal fracture left distal femur
- ▶ abnormal radiolucency in left popliteal fossa with horizontal component corresponding to clinically observed deep laceration
- ▶ fracture left proximal tibia as previously, now with periosteal reaction extending down the tibial shaft
- ▶ metaphyseal fracture left proximal fibula.

➥ The original radiographs show a vague oval-shaped radiolucency in the proximal tibia interpreted as a bone cyst. However, neither the margins of the 'cyst' nor the fracture are as sharp as would be expected following an acute injury. Furthermore, there is some periosteal reaction along the anterior and medial margins of the tibial shaft. These appearances in conjunction with the soft tissue swelling suggest a non-united (and/or infected) fracture.

➥ Notice the acute rib fractures demonstrated on the faxitron images. Their presence was initially suspected by the pathologist on gross examination of the chest.

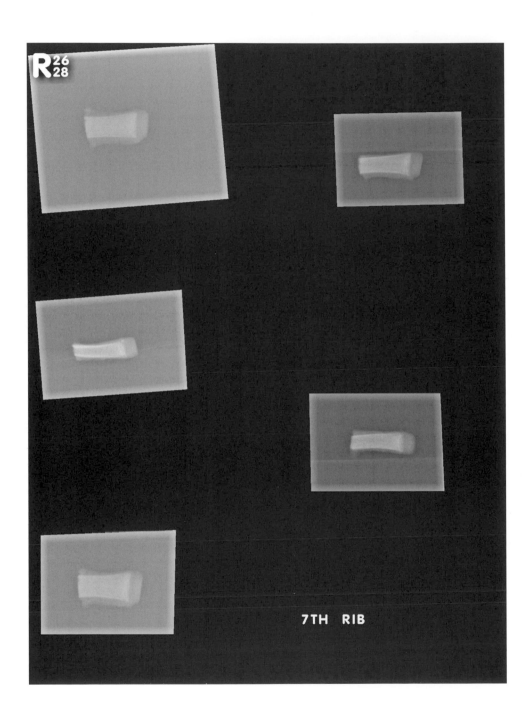

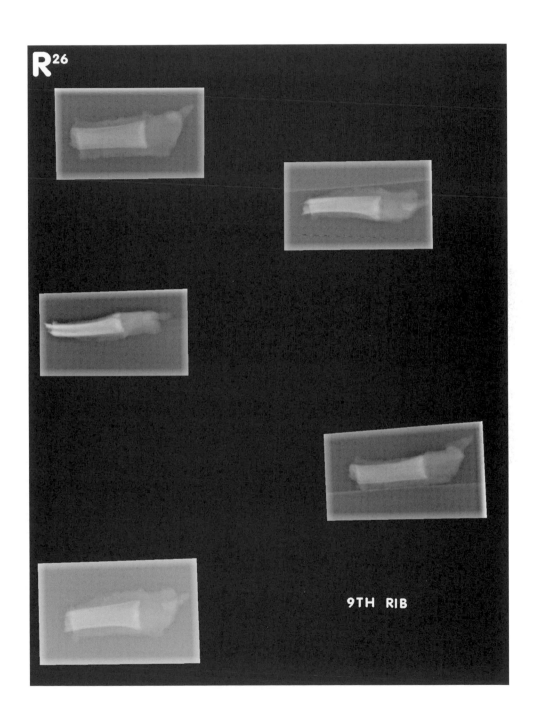

R²⁶

9TH RIB

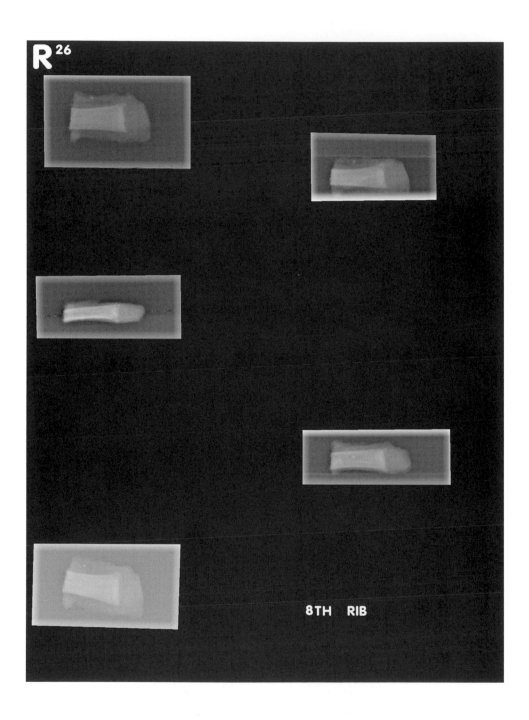

CASE 5A

History:
- ➡ 11-week-old infant with multiple facial haemangiomata
- ➡ brought into A&E with swelling and redness of the leg
- ➡ temperature 37.7 °C, blood tests normal
- ➡ the radiograph was initially reported in A&E as normal, and treatment for cellulitis was initiated
- ➡ following review by a radiologist, a skeletal survey was performed.

Radiograph right femur:
- ➡ describe the findings.

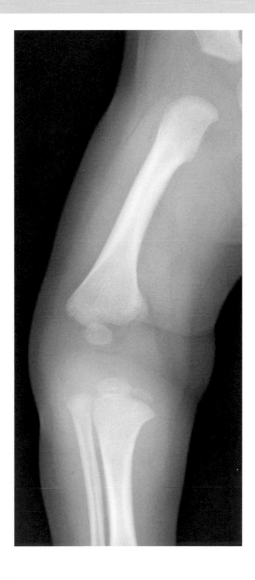

CASE 5B

➤ There are CMLs of the right distal femur and proximal tibia.

Skeletal survey:
➤ the suggested differential diagnoses were:
  ▶ osteogenesis imperfecta type IV
  ▶ congenital infection
  ▶ child abuse
➤ discuss these possibilities.

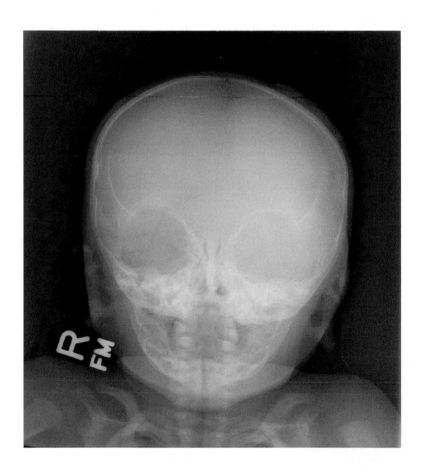

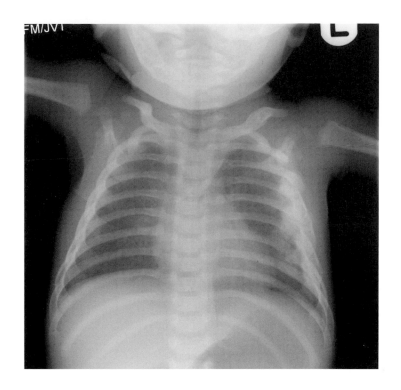

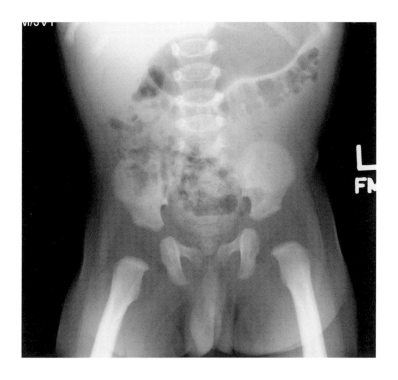

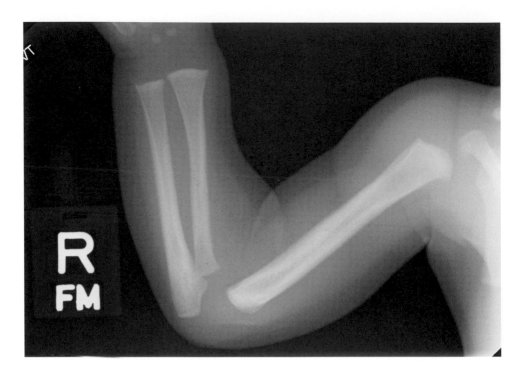

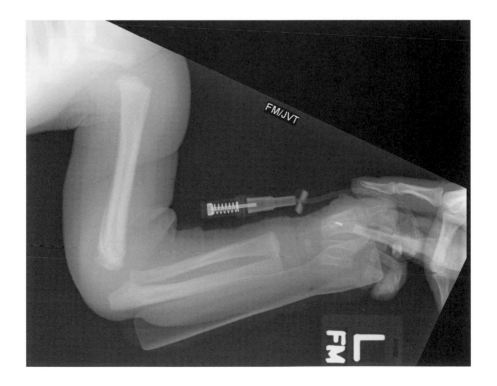

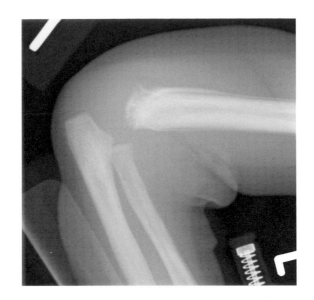

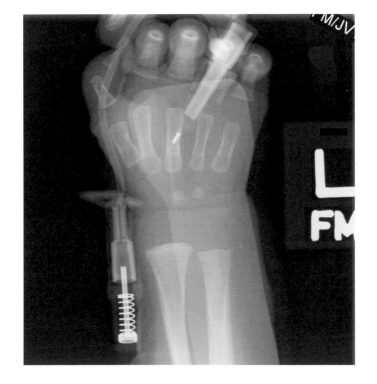

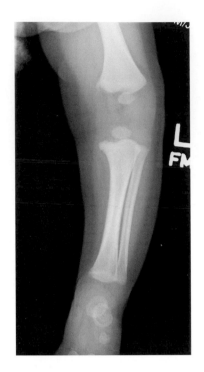

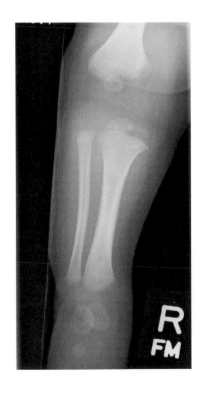

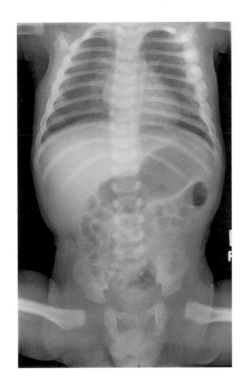

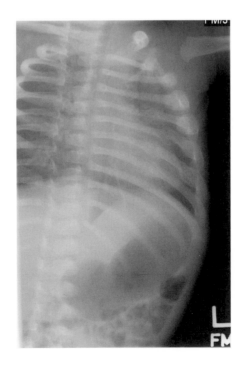

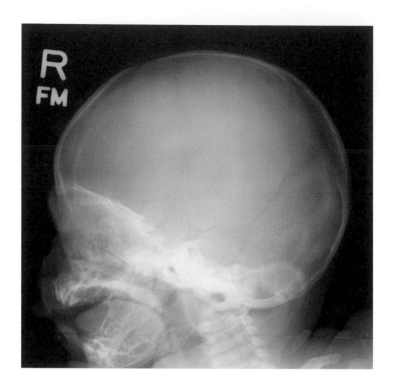

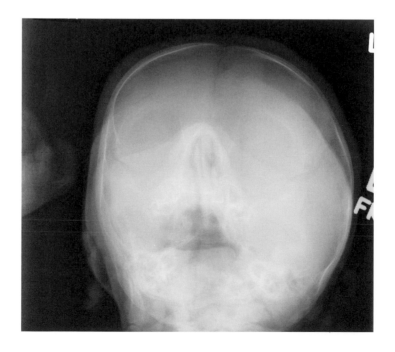

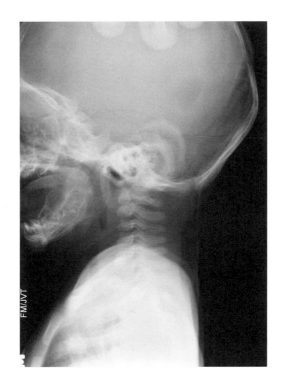

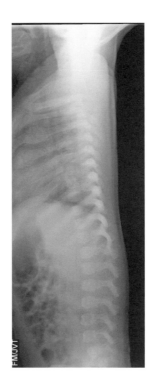

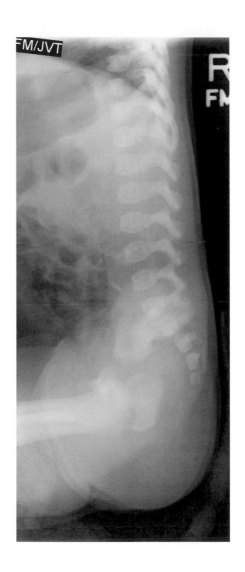

CASE 5C

➥ In all, this 11-week-old infant has the following fractures:
  ▶ left posterior ribs 4–7 (2–4 weeks old)
  ▶ left lateral ribs 2–4 (4–6 weeks old)
  ▶ CMLs right distal femur, left proximal tibia, left distal tibia (<4 weeks)
  ▶ CMLs right proximal tibia, right distal tibia, left distal femur (<4 weeks, probably <7 days)
  ▶ left clavicle (6–8 weeks old)
  ▶ left supracondylar fracture (4–6 weeks old).
➥ There are no wormian bones – which is consistent with osteogenesis imperfecta type IV. However bone density is within normal limits, the bones are not slender and CMLs are unusual in osteogenesis imperfecta.
➥ The apparent symmetry of the lesions led to a suggestion of congenital infection (the infant also had dilated ventricles but no intracranial calcification). The radiological appearances are not those of a TORCH infection. Multiple rib fractures in the context of congenital infection would be most unusual.
➥ Multiple unexplained fractures occurring on at least three separate occasions in an 11-week-old infant *must* raise the suspicion of abuse.

CASE 6A

History:
- a ten-month-old infant presented unwell with loss of appetite and diarrhoea
- examination revealed various bruises and a lump over her spine
- she appeared to be in urinary retention
- following a spine radiograph, a skeletal survey was performed.

Spinal radiograph:
- describe the abnormality – what is the likely mechanism?

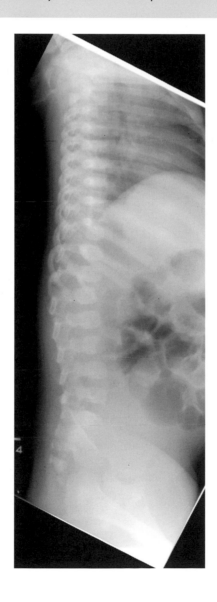

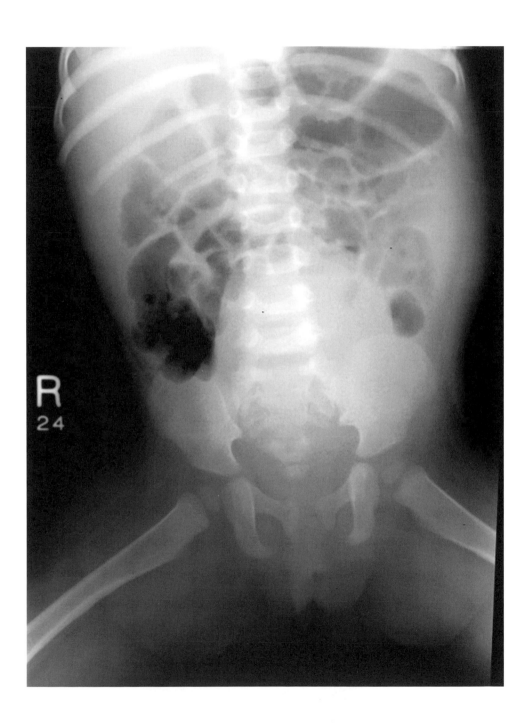

CASE 6B

- There is spondylolisthesis of T12 on L1.
- The AP radiograph demonstrates a large soft tissue density which was confirmed to be a full bladder.
- The mechanism of this injury is most likely a significant hyperflexion force – any adult carer should have been aware of the injury and/or been aware of the swelling over her back, identified by hospital staff.

Skeletal survey:
- what is the minimum number of traumatic episodes this infant has sustained?

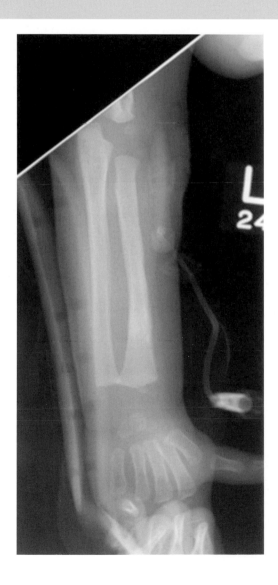

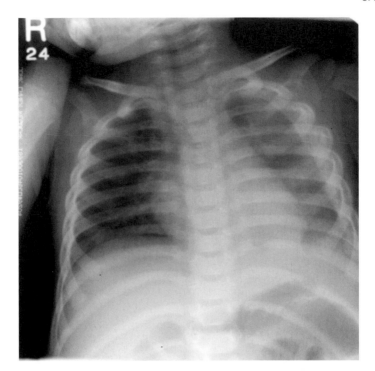

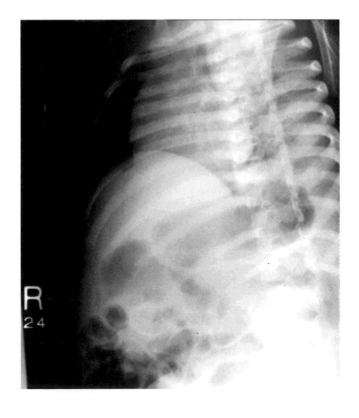

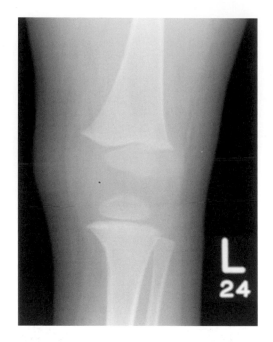

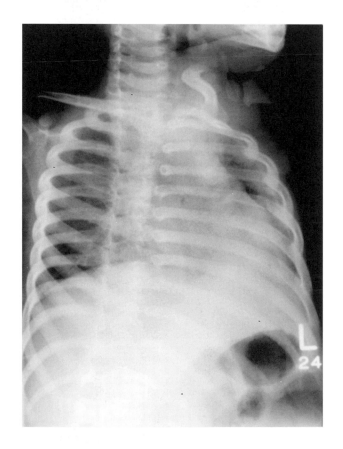

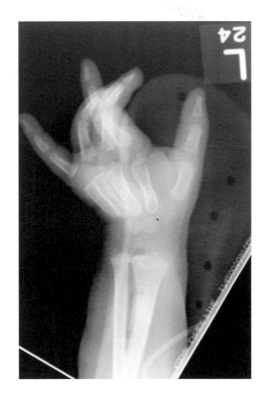

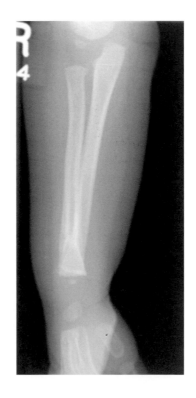

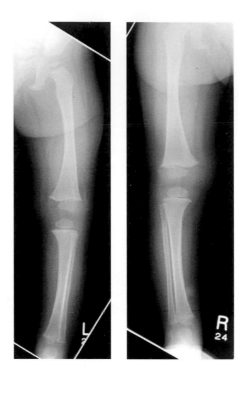

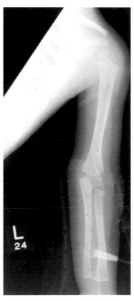

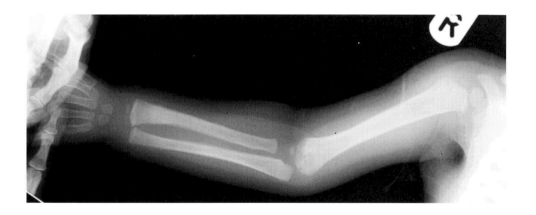

CASE 6C

➥ The injuries may be summarised as follows:
  ▶ spinal injury (<7–10 days)
  ▶ multiple rib fractures (<7–10 days)
    — note associated left pleural effusion
  ▶ multiple rib fractures (variable, 2–6 weeks)
  ▶ CML left proximal tibia (<4 weeks, probably <7 days)
  ▶ periosteal reaction distal right radius (2–4 weeks)
  ▶ periosteal reaction distal left radius and ulna (2–4 weeks).
➥ Given the multiple sites and ages of the injuries, at least four separate
  applications of force would be required.

Follow-up radiographs:
➥ i: Day 8
➥ ii: Day 15
➥ iii: Day 69.

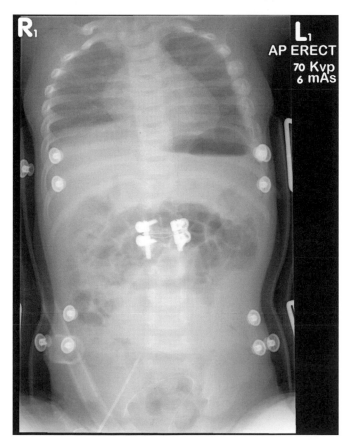

i

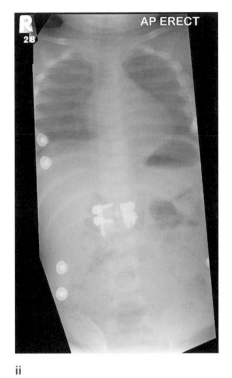

ii

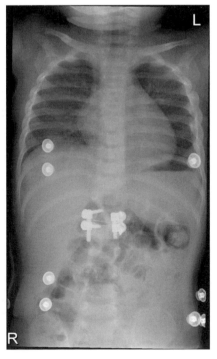

iii

CASE 7A

➡ This 3-month-old twin was taken to A&E because he was not moving his arm.

➡ A 22-month-old sibling had apparently inflicted the injury when the adult carer was temporarily away from the room.

Radiograph left arm and subsequent skeletal survey:

➡ comment on the quality of the survey

➡ what should be done next?

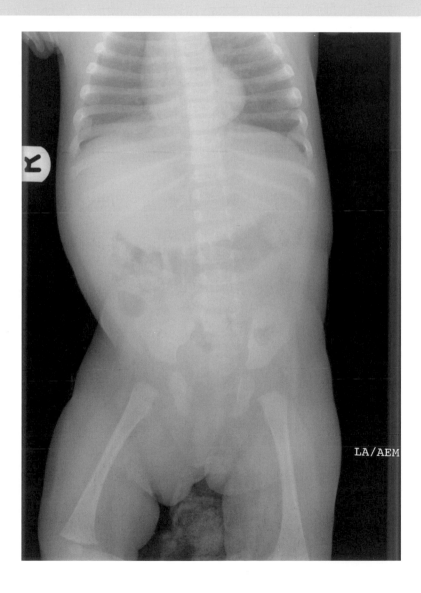

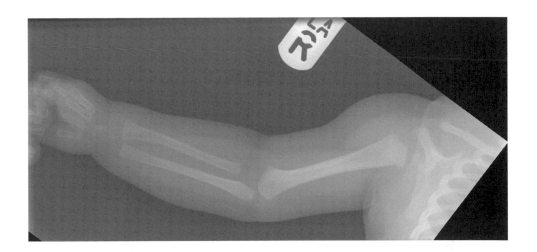

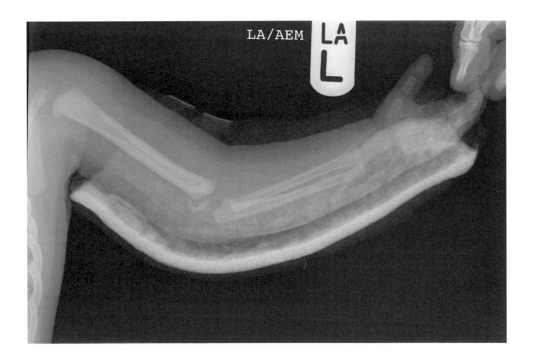

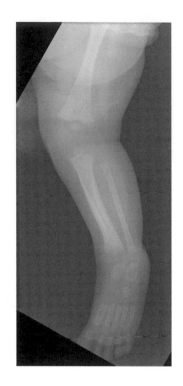

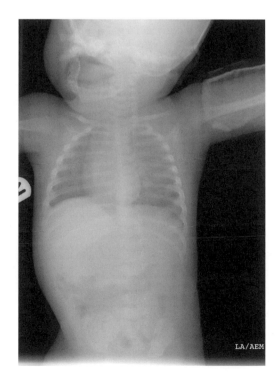

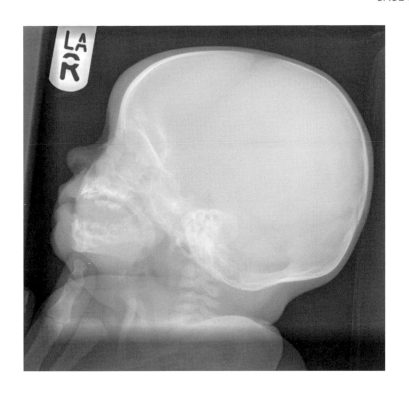

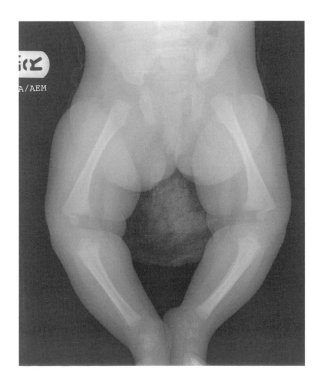

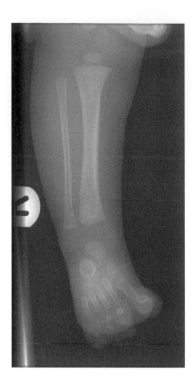

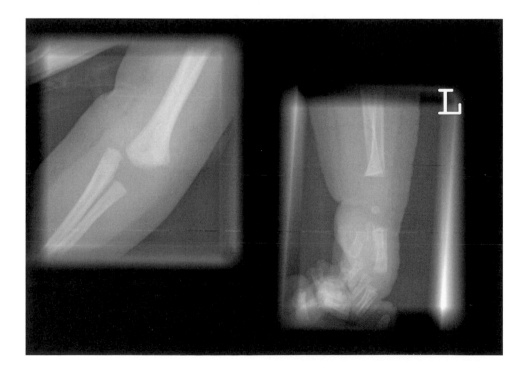

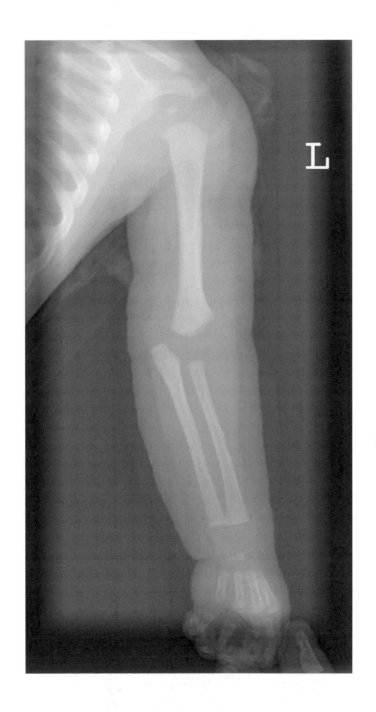

CASE 7B

➥ Multiple fractures:
  ▶ left supracondylar (<7–10 days)
  ▶ CML right distal tibia (<4 weeks)
  ▶ fractures lateral left 6th and 7th ribs (>8 weeks).
➥ All radiographs obtained as part of the skeletal survey performed by the referring hospital have been presented. This does not conform to the BSPR guidelines[8] and babygrams should never be performed in the context of suspected abuse.[7,8,11]
➥ Skeletal surveys of the twin and 22-month-old sibling should now be performed.

Skeletal surveys:
➥ i: 22-month-old sibling
➥ ii: 3-month-old twin.

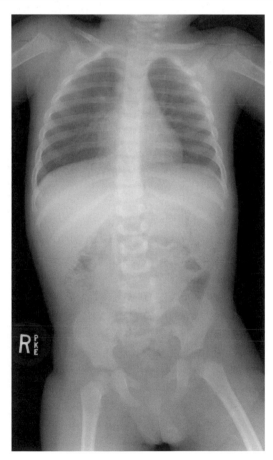

i

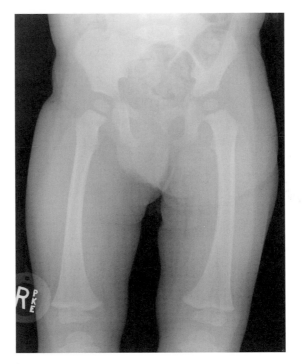

i

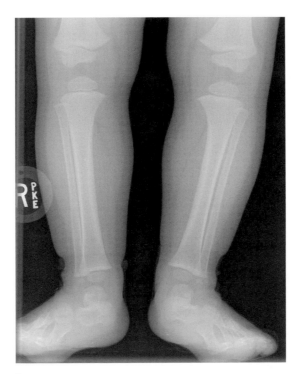

i

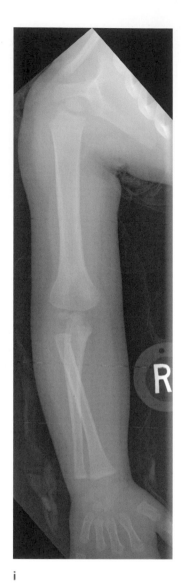

i

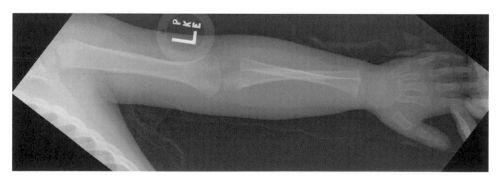

i

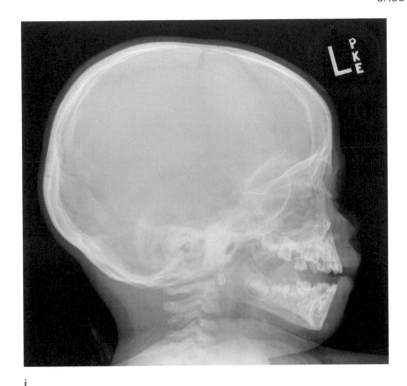

i

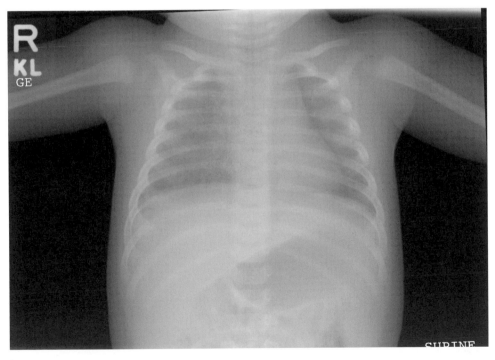

i

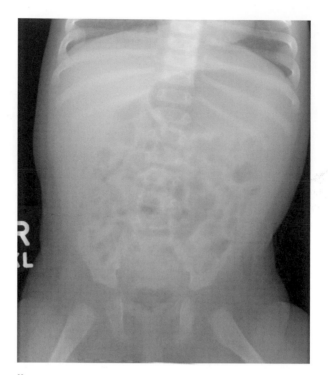

ii

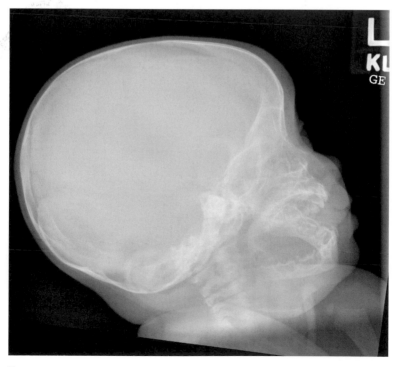

ii

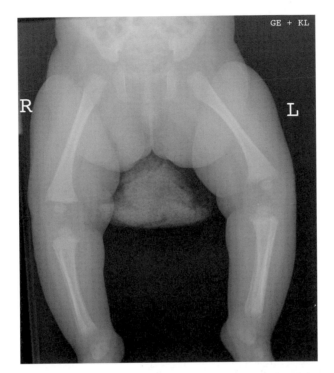

ii

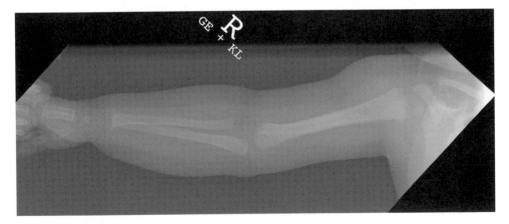

ii

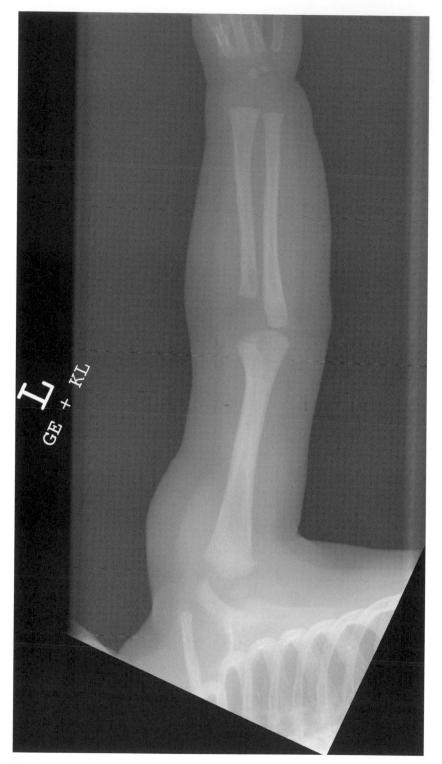

ii

CASE 7C

- ➡ A: Normal (although limited) survey in the 22-month-old sibling.
- ➡ B: The 3-month-old twin also had CMLs of the right proximal humerus, right distal femur, left proximal tibia, left distal tibia and possibly left proximal humerus (all <4 weeks old).

CASE 8A

➥ Five-month-old infant not using his left arm.
➥ No past or family history of note.
➥ Radiographs of both arms obtained.

Arm radiographs:
➥ issue a report for this examination.

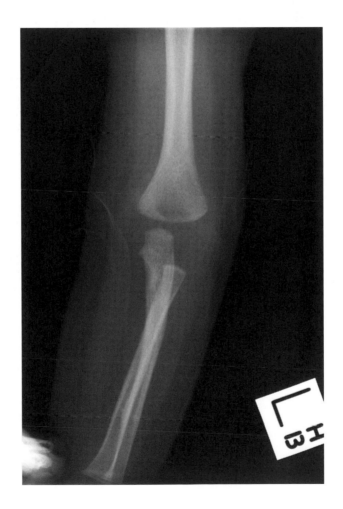

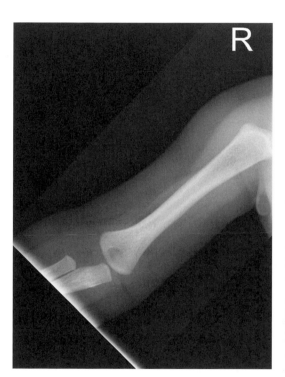

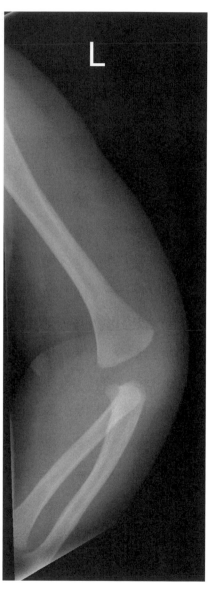

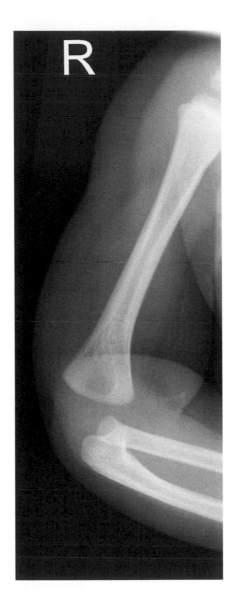

CASE 8B

➥ There is soft tissue swelling on the left with a centrally placed capitellum (compare to the normal right side), indicating fracture/dislocation.
➥ The right side is normal.

Comments:

➥ malposition of the capitellum was not identified on initial interpretation
➥ traction was applied for a presumed pulled elbow and imaging was repeated on Day 3
➥ as a result of the findings a skeletal survey was performed.

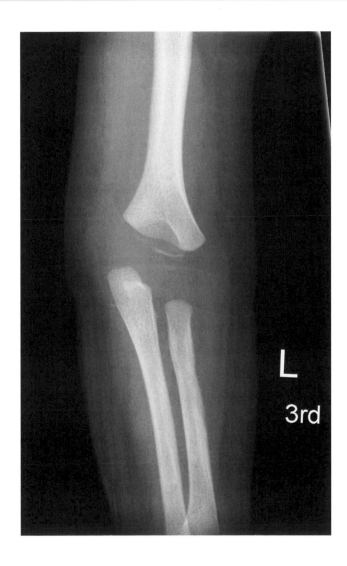

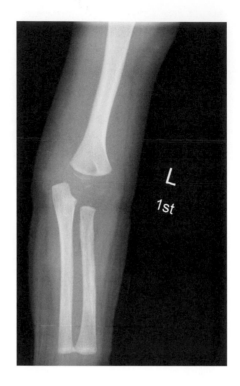

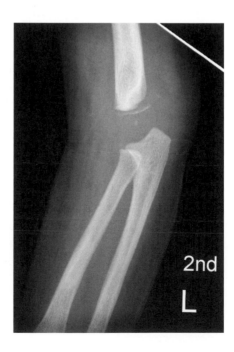

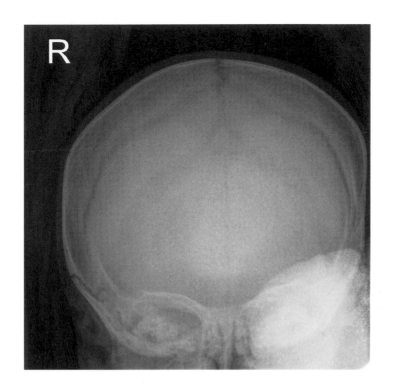

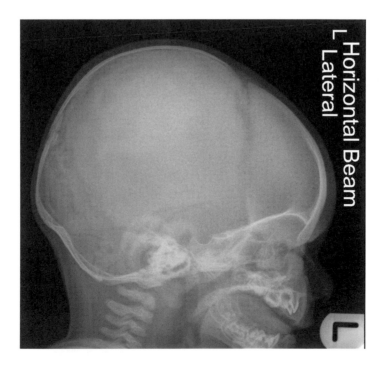

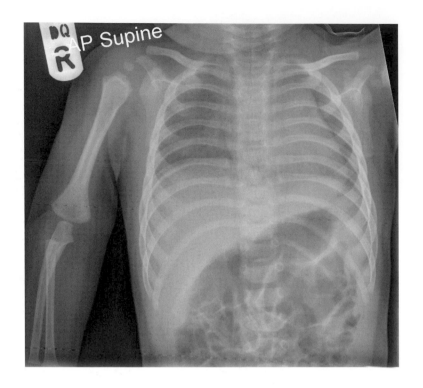

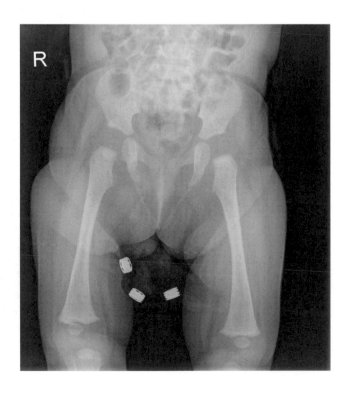

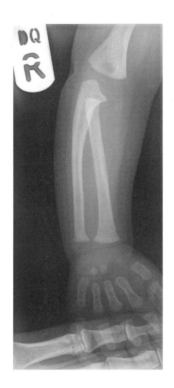

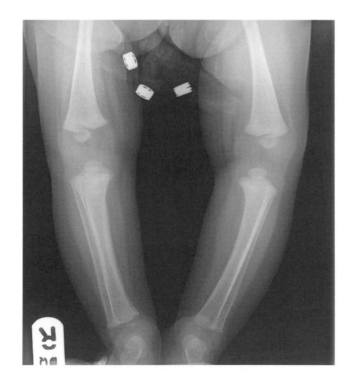

CASE 8C

➥ The following injuries are identified:
  ▶ left distal humeral transcondylar fracture (<7–10 days)
  ▶ CML right distal femur (<4 weeks)
  ▶ CML right distal tibia (<4 weeks)
  ▶ periosteal reaction right tibia (at least 2 weeks).

Comments:
➥ legal representatives considered that the distal humeral fracture may have been caused by medical professionals as they attempted to reduce the presumed pulled elbow
➥ this is highly unlikely, and would not explain the clinical and radiological signs at initial presentation, and obviously does not explain the other injuries
➥ regardless of the cause of the distal humeral fracture, given the other injuries, this child had clearly been a victim of physical abuse.

CASE 9A

History:

➡ four-month-old infant brought in following sudden unexpected death.

Skeletal survey prior to post-mortem:

➡ issue a report.

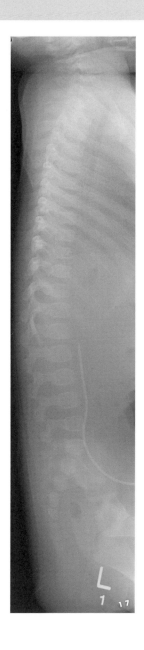

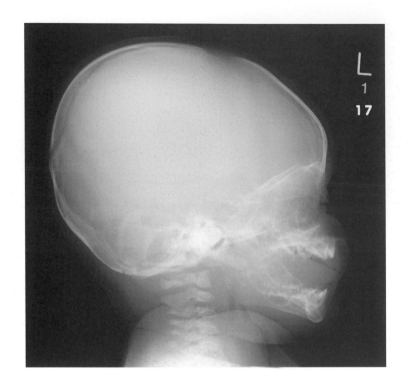

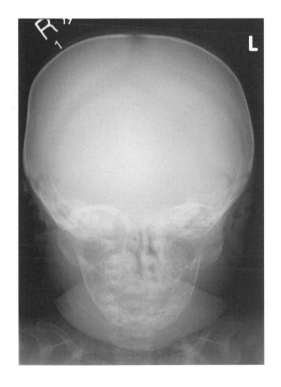

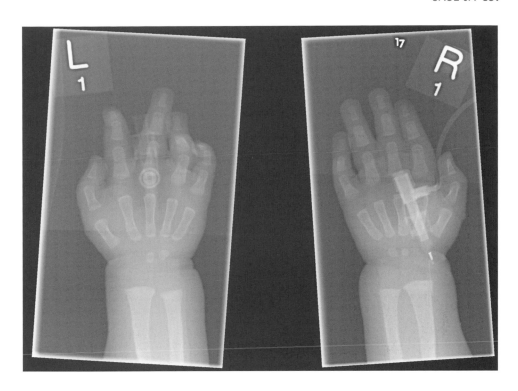

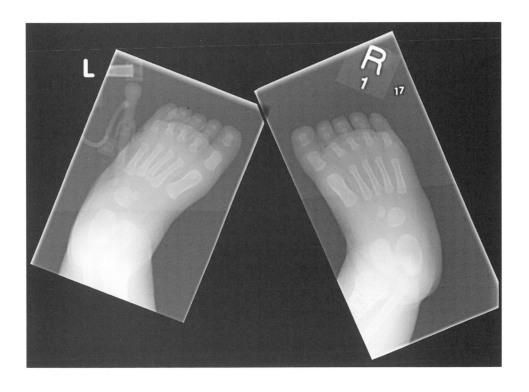

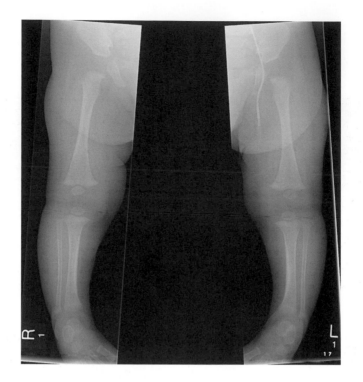

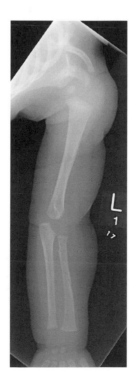

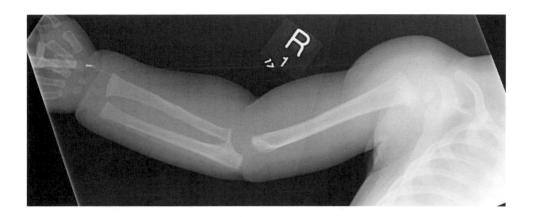

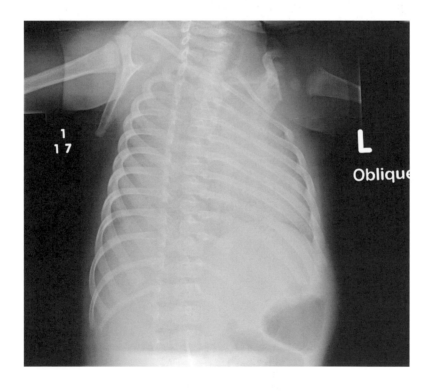

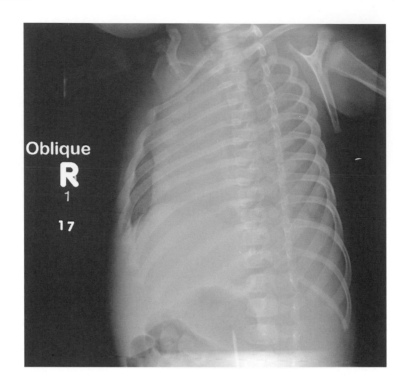

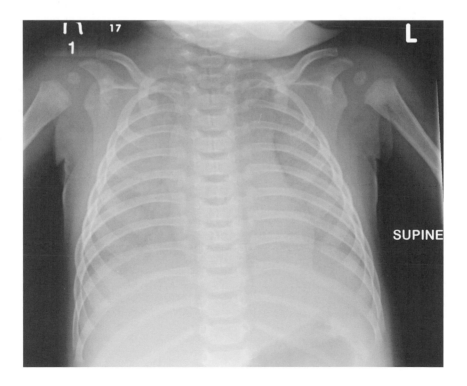

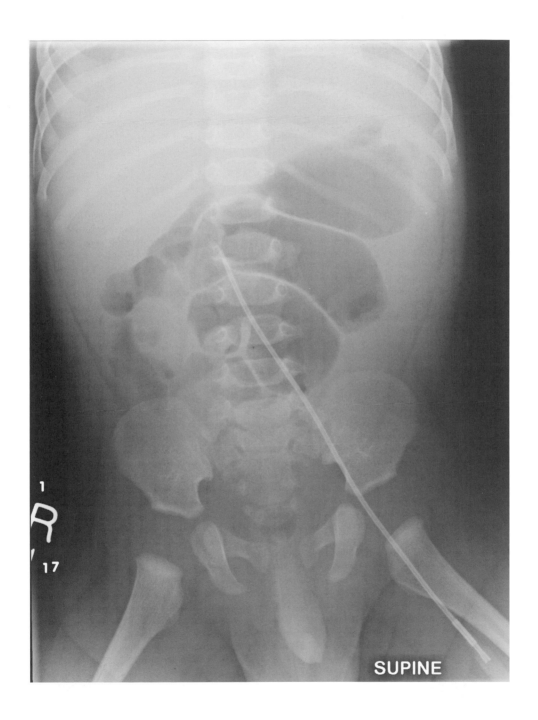

SUPINE

CASE 9B

→ There is widening of the cranial sutures which may be normal in infants or indicate raised intracranial pressure.
  ▶ CT head performed as a routine investigation in suspected abuse revealed generalised brain swelling and oedema and an acute subdural haemorrhage (strongly indicative of abuse).
→ The survey is otherwise normal.

Gross pathological examination identified acute rib fractures, and faxitron images of the excised ribs were obtained.

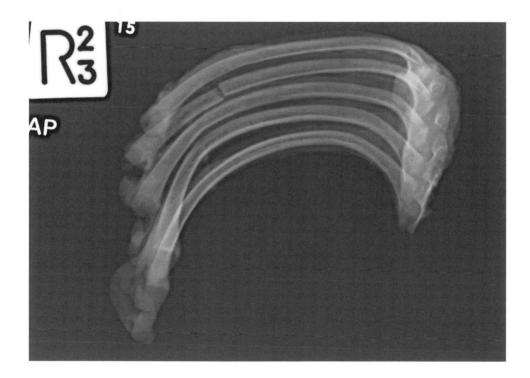

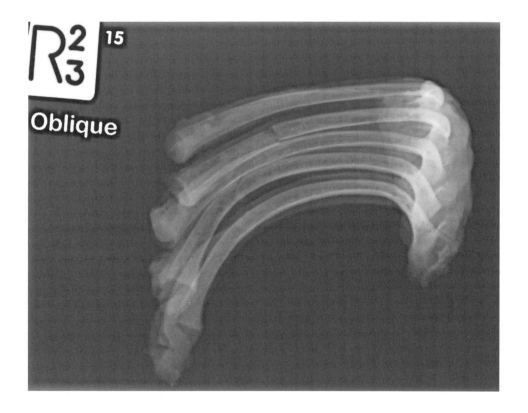

CASE 9C

➡ Post-mortem examination found acute fractures of the right 5th–7th ribs.
➡ Faxitron confirmed the acute fracture of the right 5th rib, but not the others.
➡ Even with the benefit of this information, the fractures cannot be identified on the chest radiographs.

Comment:
➡ it is well known that radiography misses acute rib fractures, and it is for this reason that follow-up radiographs are advised in surviving victims of abuse.[10]

CASE 10A

History:
➡ 33-day-old infant brought in with unexplained swelling of her right femur
➡ no past medical or family history of note.

Right femur and skeletal survey:
➡ comment on the imaging.

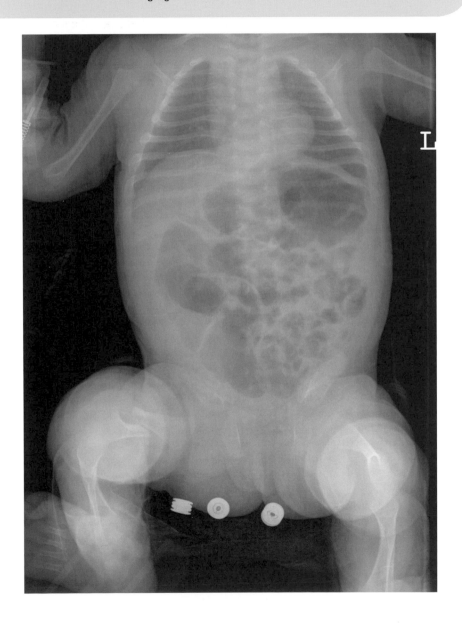

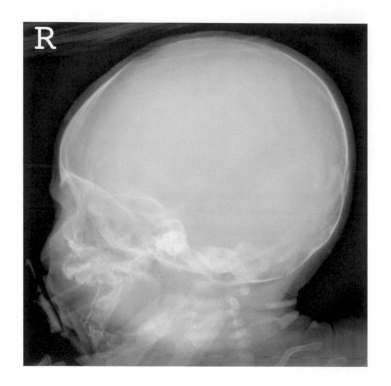

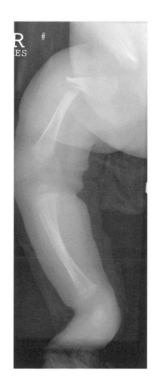

CASE 10B

- ➥ Inadequate skeletal survey. DO NOT exclude any metaphyseal fractures on the basis of this examination.
- ➥ No wormian bones visible on the skull radiograph.

Further imaging (Day 33):
- ➥ report on the radiographs.

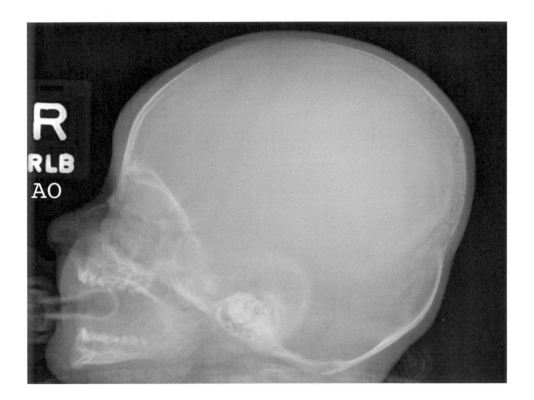

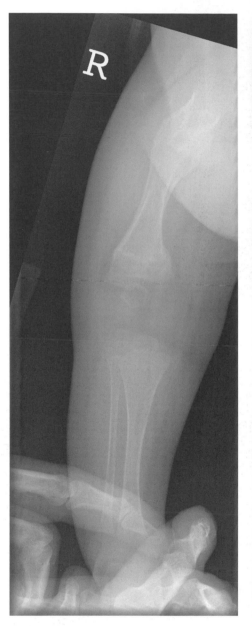
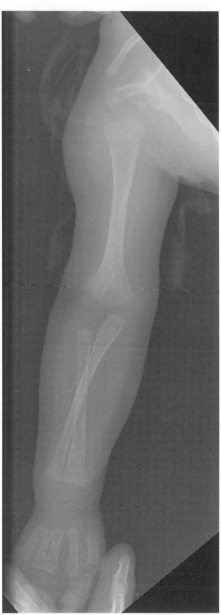

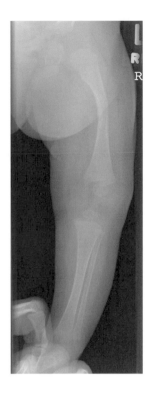

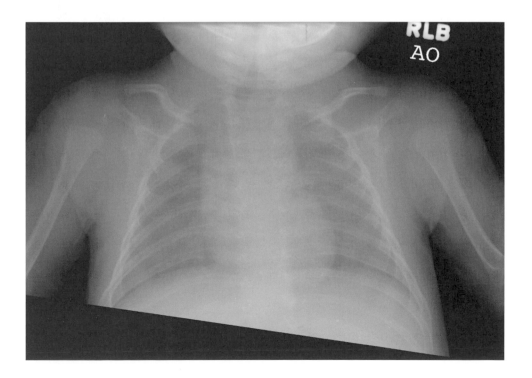

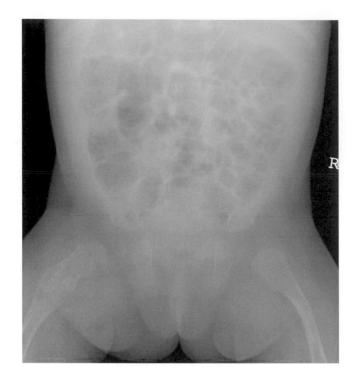

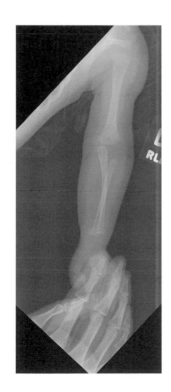

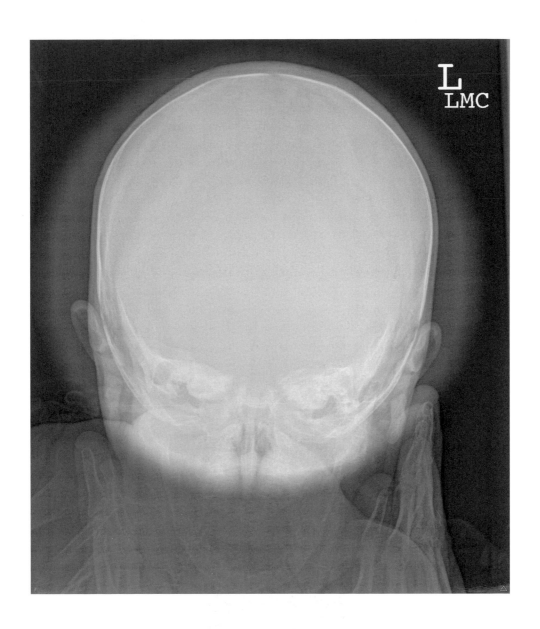

CASE 10C

- ➥ Healing fracture right proximal femur.
- ➥ Impacted fracture right distal femur (<7–10 days).
- ➥ Bowing left femur.
- ➥ Multiple wormian bones:
  - ▶ best seen on the Towne's projection.

Comments:
- ➥ notice how the obliquity of the initial lateral skull radiograph obscures the wormian bones
- ➥ this infant has osteogenesis imperfecta, probably type IV – radiographic findings are perhaps a little too severe for type I (*see* Plate 9.5).

1   Silverman FN. Unrecognised trauma in infants, the battered child syndrome, and the syndrome of Ambroise Tardieu [Rigler lecture]. *Radiology.* 1972; **104**: 337–53.

2   Caffey J. Multiple fractures in the long bones of infants suffering from chronic subdural hematoma. *Am J Roentgenol.* 1946; **56**: 163–73.

3   Richman HA. From a radiologist's judgement to public policy on child abuse and neglect: what have we wrought? *Pediatr Radiol.* 2000; **30**: 219–28.

4   McClain PW, Sacks JJ, Froehlke RG, *et al.* Estimates of fatal child abuse and neglect, United States, 1979 through 1988. *Pediatrics.* 1993; **91**: 338–43.

5   Kleinman PK, Marks SC Jr, Richmond JM, *et al.* Inflicted skeletal injury: a post-mortem radiologic-histopathologic study in 31 infants. *Am J Roentgenol.* 1995; **165**: 647–50.

6   Kemp AM, Butler A, Morris S, *et al.* Which radiological investigations should be performed to identify fractures in suspected child abuse? *Clin Radiol.* 2006; **61**: 723–36.

7   Offiah AC, Hall CM. Observational study of skeletal surveys in suspected non-accidental injury. *Clin Radiol.* 2003; **58**: 702–5.

8   British Society of Paediatric Radiologists. *Standard for skeletal surveys in suspected non-accidental injury (NAI) in children.* Available at: www.bspr.org.uk/nai.htm (accessed 12 March 2009).

9   Swinson S, Tapp M, Brindley R, *et al.* An audit of skeletal surveys for suspected non-accidental injury following publication of the British Society of Paediatric Radiology guidelines. *Clin Radiol.* 2008; **63**: 651–6.

10 Kleinman PK, Nimkin K, Spevak MR, *et al.* Follow-up skeletal surveys in suspected child abuse. *Am J Roentgenol.* 1996; **167**: 893–6.

11 American College of Radiology. *Practice Guideline for Skeletal Surveys in Children* 1997 (Res. 22) Revised 2001 (Res. 31) Revised 2006 (Res. 47,17,35). Available at: www.acr.org/SecondaryMainMenuCategories/quality_safety/guidelines/pediatric/skeletal_surveys.aspx (accessed 12 March 2009).

12 Jaspan T, Griffiths PD, McConachie NS, *et al.* Neuroimaging for non-accidental injury in childhood: a proposed protocol. *Clin Radiol.* 2003; **58**: 44–53.

13 Ng CS, Hall CM. Costochondral junction fractures and intra-abdominal trauma in non-accidental injury (child abuse). *Pediatr Radiol.* 1998; **28**: 671–6.

14 The Royal College of Pathologists. *Guidelines on autopsy practice: report of a working group of the Royal College of Pathologists.* Appendix 7: Guidelines for autopsy investigation in post-neonatal infant deaths or sudden unexpected deaths in infancy; 2002. Available at: www.rcpath.org/resources/pdf/appendix_7.pdf (accessed 12 March 2009)

15 Sonoda M, Takano M, Miyahara J, *et al.* Computed radiography utilizing scanning laser stimulated luminescence. *Radiology.* 1983; **148**: 833–8.

16 Kangarloo H, Boechat MI, Barbaric Z, *et al.* Two-year clinical experience with a computed radiography system. *Am J Roentgenol.* 1988; **151**: 605–8.

17 Shaw G. A clinician's guide to digital X-ray systems. *J R Soc Med.* 2001; **94**: 391–5.

18 Chotas HG, Ravin CE. Digital chest radiography with a solid-state flat-panel X-ray detector: contrast-detail evaluation with processed images processed on film hard copy. *Radiology.* 2001; **218**: 679–82.

19 Schaefer-Prokop CM, Prokop M. Storage phosphor radiography. *Eur Radiol.* 1997; **7**(Suppl 3): S58–S65.

20 Cowen AR, Workman A, Price JS. Physical aspects of photostimulable phosphor computed radiography. *Br J Radiol.* 1993; **66**: 332–45.

21 Offiah AC, Hall CM. Evaluation of the Community of European Communities quality criteria for the paediatric lateral spine. *Br J Radiol.* 2003; **76**: 885–90.

22 Offiah AC, Moon L, Hall CM, *et al.* Diagnostic accuracy of fracture detection in suspected non-accidental injury: effect of edge enhancement and digital display on observer performance. *Clin Radiol.* 2006; **61**: 163–73.

23 Kogutt MS, Swischuk LE, Fagan CJ. Patterns of injury and significance of uncommon fractures in the battered child syndrome. *Am J Roentgenol Radium Ther Nucl Med.* 1974; **121**: 143–9.

24   Lauer B, ten Broeck ET, Grossman M. Battered child syndrome: review of 130 patients with controls. *Pediatrics*. 1974; **54**: 67–70.

25   Akbarnia BA, Akbarnia NO. The role of the orthopedist in child abuse and neglect. *Orthop Clin North Am*. 1976; **7**: 733–42.

26   Galleno H, Oppenheim WL. The battered child syndrome revisited. *Clin Orthop Relat Res*. 1982; **162**: 11–19.

27   O'Neill JA Jr, Meacham WF, Griffin JP, *et al*. Patterns of injury in the battered child syndrome. *J Trauma*. 1973; **13**: 332–9.

28   Mathew MO, Ramamohan N, Bennet GC. Importance of bruising associated with paediatric fractures: prospective observational study. *BMJ*. 1998; **317**: 1117–18.

29   Carpenter RF. The prevalence and distribution of bruising in babies. *Arch Dis Child*. 1999; **80**: 363–6.

30   Roberton DM, Barbor P, Hull D. Unusual injury? Recent injury in normal children and children with suspected non-accidental injury. *BMJ* (Clin Res Ed). 1982; **285**: 1399–401.

31   Rao P, Carty H. Non-accidental injury: review of the radiology. *Clin Radiol*. 1999; **54**: 11–24.

32   Chapman S. The radiological dating of injuries. *Arch Dis Child*. 1992; **67**: 1063–5.

33   McMahon P, Grossman W, Gaffney M, *et al*. Soft tissue injury as an indication of child abuse. *J Bone Joint Surg Am*. 1995; **77**: 1179–83.

34   Kleinman PK, Belanger PL, Karellas A, *et al*. Normal metaphyseal radiologic variants not to be confused with findings of infant abuse. *Am J Roentgenol*. 1991; **156**: 781–3.

35   Carty H. Differentiation of child abuse from osteogenesis imperfecta. *Am J Roentgenol*. 1991; **156**: 635–6.

36   Carty H. Case report: Child abuse – necklace calcification – a sign of strangulation. *Br J Radiol*. 1993; **66**: 1186–8.

37   Worlock P, Stower M, Barbor P. Patterns of fractures in accidental and non-accidental injury in children: a comparative study. *BMJ* (Clin Res Ed). 1986; **293**: 100–2.

38   Loder RT, Bookout C. Fracture patterns in battered children. *J Orthop Trauma*. 1991; **5**: 428–33.

39   Carty H, Pierce A. Non-accidental injury: a retrospective analysis of a large cohort. *Eur Radiol*. 2002; **1**: 2919–25.

40   Merten DF, Radkowski MA, Leonidas JC. The abused child: a radiological reappraisal. *Radiology*. 1983; **146**: 377–81.

41   Carty H. Fractures caused by child abuse. *J Bone Joint Surg Br*. 1993; **75**: 849–57.

42   Caffey J. The parent-infant traumatic stress syndrome (Caffey-Kempe syndrome) (Battered babe syndrome) [The first annual Neuhauser presidential address of the Society for Paediatric Radiology]. *Am J Roentgenol Radium Ther Nucl Med*. 1972; **114**: 217–19.

43   Leonidas J. Skeletal trauma in the child abuse syndrome. *Pediatr Ann*. 1983; **12**: 875–1.

44   Kleinman PK. Diagnostic imaging in infant abuse. *Am J Roentgenol*. 1990; **155**: 703–12.

45   Kleinman PK. Skeletal trauma: general considerations. In: Kleinman PK, editor. *Diagnostic Imaging of Child Abuse*. 2nd ed. St Louis, MO: Mosby Inc.; 1998. Chapter 2 pp. 8–25.

46   Astley R. Multiple metaphyseal fractures in small children (metaphyseal fragility of bone). *Br J Radiol*. 1953; **26**: 577–83.

47   Kleinman PK, Marks SC Jr, Blackbourne B. The metaphyseal lesion in abused infants: a radiologic-histopathologic study. *Am J Roentgenol*. 1986; **146**: 895–905.

48   Kleinman PK, Marks SC Jr. A regional approach to the classic metaphyseal lesion in abused infants: the proximal tibia. *Am J Roentgenol*. 1996; **166**: 421–6.

49   Kleinman PK, Marks SC Jr. A regional approach to the classic metaphyseal lesion in abused infants: the distal tibia. *Am J Roentgenol*. 1996; **166**: 1207–12.

50   Kleinman PK, Marks SC Jr. A regional approach to the classic metaphyseal lesion in abused infants: the proximal humerus. *Am J Roentgenol*. 1996; **167**: 1399–403.

51   Kleinman PK, Marks SC Jr. A regional approach to the classic metaphyseal lesion in abused infants: the distal femur. *Am J Roentgenol*. 1998; **170**: 43–7.

52   Cramer KE. Orthopedic aspects of child abuse. *Pediatr Clin North Am*. 1996; **43**: 1035–51.

53   King J, Diefendorf D, Apthorp J, *et al*. Analysis of 429 fractures in 189 battered children. *J Pediatr Orthop*. 1988; **8**: 585–9.

54   Drvaric DM, Morrell SM, Wyly JB, *et al*. Fracture patterns in the battered child syndrome. *J South Orthop Assoc*. 1992; **1**: 20–5.

55 Scherl SA, Miller L, Lively N, *et al.* Accidental and non-accidental femur fractures in children. *Clin Orthop.* 2000; **376**: 96–105.

56 McClelland CQ, Heiple KG. Fractures in the first year of life: a diagnostic dilemma. *Am J Dis Child.* 1982; **136**: 26–9.

57 Herndon WA. Child abuse in a military population. *J Pediatr Orthop.* 1983; **3**: 73–6.

58 Strait RT, Siegel RM, Shapiro RA. Humeral fractures without obvious etiologies in children less than 3 years of age: when is it abuse? *Pediatrics.* 1995; **96**: 667–71.

59 Anderson WA. The significance of femoral fractures in children. *Ann Emerg Med.* 1982; **11**: 174–7.

60 Beals RK, Tufts E. Fractured femur in infancy: the role of child abuse. *J Pediatr Orthop.* 1983; **3**: 583–6.

61 Thomas SA, Rosenfield NS, Leventhal JM, *et al.* Long-bone fractures in young children: distinguishing accidental injuries from child abuse. *Pediatrics.* 1991; **88**: 471–6.

62 Leventhal JM, Thomas SA, Rosenfield NS, *et al.* Fractures in young children: distinguishing child abuse from unintentional injuries. *Am J Dis Child.* 1993; **147**: 87–92.

63 Boal DK, Felman AH, Krugman RD. Controversial aspects of child abuse: a roundtable discussion. *Pediatr Radiol.* 2001; **31**: 760–4.

64 Johnstone AJ, Zuberi SH, Scobie WG. Skull fractures in children: a population study. *J Accid Emerg Med.* 1996; **13**: 386–9.

65 Hobbs CJ. Skull fracture and the diagnosis of child abuse. *Arch Dis Child.* 1984; **59**: 246–52.

66 Helfer RE, Slovis TL, Black M. Injuries resulting when small children fall out of bed. *Pediatrics.* 1977; **60**: 533–5.

67 Nimityongskul P, Anderson LD. The likelihood of injuries when children fall out of bed. *J Pediatr Orthop.* 1987; **7**: 184–6.

68 Chapman S. Radiological aspects of non-accidental injury. *J R Soc Med.* 1990; **83**: 67–71.

69 Chiaviello CT, Christoph RA, Bond GR. Stairway-related injuries in children. *Pediatrics.* 1994; **94**: 679–81.

70 Joffe M, Ludwig S. Stairway injuries in children. *Pediatrics.* 1988; **82**: 457–61.

71 Lloyd DA, Carty H, Patterson M, *et al.* Predictive value of skull radiography for intracranial injury in children with blunt head injury. *Lancet.* 1997; **349**: 821–4.

72 Saulsbury FT, Alford BA. Intracranial bleeding from child abuse: the value of skull radiographs. *Pediatr Radiol.* 1982; **12**: 175–8.

73 Lis EF, Frauenberger GS. Multiple fractures associated with subdural hematoma in infancy. *Pediatrics.* 1950; **6**: 890–2.

74 Woolley PV Jr, Evans WA Jr. Significance of skeletal lesions in infants resembling those of traumatic origin. *JAMA.* 1955; **158**: 539–43.

75 Feldman KW, Brewer DK. Child abuse, cardiopulmonary resuscitation and rib fractures. *Pediatrics.* 1984; **73**: 339–42.

76 Bush CM, Jones JS, Cohle SD, *et al.* Paediatric injuries from cardiopulmonary resuscitation. *Ann Emerg Med.* 1996; **28**: 40–4.

77 Bulloch B, Schubert CJ, Brophy PD, *et al.* Cause and clinical characteristics of rib fractures in infants. *Pediatrics.* 2000; **105**: e48. Available at: http://pediatrics.aappublications.org/cgi/content/full/105/4/e48 (accessed 27 Feb 2009).

78 Chalumeau M, Foix-L'Helias L, Scheinmann P, *et al.* Rib fractures after chest physiotherapy for bronchiolitis or pneumonia in infants. *Pediatr Radiol.* 2002; **32**: 644–7.

79 Thomas PS. Rib fractures in infancy. *Ann Radiol.* 1977; **20**: 115–22.

80 Levine MG, Holroyde J, Woods JR Jr, *et al.* Birth trauma: incidence and predisposing factors. *Obstet Gynecol.* 1984; **63**: 792–5.

81 Spevak MR, Kleinman PK, Belanger PL, *et al.* Cardiopulmonary resuscitation and rib fractures in infants: a post-mortem radiologic-pathologic study. *JAMA.* 1994; **272**: 617–18.

82 Kleinman PK, Marks SC Jr, Nimkin K, *et al.* Rib fractures in 31 abused infants: post-mortem radiologic-histopathologic study. *Radiology.* 1996; **200**: 807–10.

83 Kwon DS, Spevak MR, Fletcher K, *et al.* Physiologic subperiosteal new bone formation: prevalence, distribution and thickness in neonates and infants. *Am J Roentgenol.* 2002; **179**: 985–8.

84 O'Connor JF, Cohen J. Dating fractures. In: Kleinman PK, editor. *Diagnostic Imaging of Child Abuse.* 2nd ed. St Louis, MO: Mosby Inc.; 1998. Chapter 7 pp. 168–77.

85 Kleinman PK, Marks SC Jr, Spevak MR, *et al.* Extension of growth-plate cartilage into the metaphysis: a sign of healing fracture in abused infants. *Am J Roentgenol.* 1991; **156**: 775–9.

86 Kleinman PK. Bony thoracic trauma. In: Kleinman PK, editor. *Diagnostic Imaging of Child Abuse.* 2nd ed. St Louis, MO: Mosby Inc.; 1998. Chapter 5 pp. 110–48.

87 Prosser I, Maguire S, Harrison SK, *et al.* How old is the fracture? Radiologic dating of fractures in children: a systematic review. *Am J Roentgenol.* 2005; **184**: 1282–6.

88 Cooper A, Floyd T, Barlow B, *et al.* Major blunt abdominal trauma due to child abuse. *J Trauma.* 1988; **28**: 1483–7.

89 Sivit CJ, Taylor GA, Eichelberger MR. Visceral injury in battered children: a changing perspective. *Radiology.* 1989; **173**: 659–1.

90 Ledbetter DJ, Hatch EI Jr, Feldman KW, *et al.* Diagnostic and surgical implications of child abuse. *Arch Surg.* 1988; **123**: 1101–5.

91 Fenton LZ, Sirotnak AP, Handler MH. Parietal pseudofracture and spontaneous intracranial hemorrhage suggesting non-accidental trauma: report of 2 cases. *Pediatr Neurosurg.* 2000; **33**: 318–22.

Index